HEALTH DISCLOSURE

The Sequence to Obesity & Disease

ADAM MASTERS

BALBOA
PRESS
A DIVISION OF HAY HOUSE

Balboa Press books may be ordered through booksellers or by contacting:

Balboa Press
A Division of Hay House
1663 Liberty Drive
Bloomington, IN 47403
www.balboapress.com
1 (877) 407-4847

Because of the dynamic nature of the Internet, any web addresses or links contained in this book may have changed since publication and may no longer be valid. The views expressed in this work are solely those of the author and do not necessarily reflect the views of the publisher, and the publisher hereby disclaims any responsibility for them.

The author of this book does not dispense medical advice or prescribe the use of any technique as a form of treatment for physical, emotional, or medical problems without the advice of a physician, either directly or indirectly. The intent of the author is only to offer information of a general nature to help you in your quest for emotional and spiritual well-being. In the event you use any of the information in this book for yourself, which is your constitutional right, the author and the publisher assume no responsibility for your actions.

Any people depicted in stock imagery provided by Thinkstock are models, and such images are being used for illustrative purposes only.
Certain stock imagery © Thinkstock.

Printed in the United States of America.

ISBN: 978-1-4525-8503-1 (sc)
ISBN: 978-1-4525-8505-5 (hc)
ISBN: 978-1-4525-8504-8 (e)

Library of Congress Control Number: 2013919467

Balboa Press rev. date: 10/30/2013

CONTENTS

INTRODUCTION
Health Disclosure

In the United States, citizens are the most doped up nation in the history of the planet. A survey conducted by the Mayo Clinic found that 70% of all Americans are on at least one prescription drug. An astounding 20% of all Americans are on at least five prescription drugs. There are a lot of books written on the subject of health, but true health is elusive to more than 90% of the population and general health is quickly eroding for all, and at a younger age. Health has the attention of a growing number of the population. There is evidence that health and aging are a source of fear in society with one American going bankrupt every second getting sick and unable to pay a healthcare bill. 50% of the population in the US has chronic illness and it eats up an incredible 18% of GDP. Give me a hospital and let's clear 90% out, it's that easy. One doctor for hormones and one doctor for autoimmune and we could point to a day on the calendar for each patient. The cure for every disease has been found with over 97% of drugs irrelevant. If you weren't born with it, you don't need to die with it.

The trouble with the health care system is that it is driven by profit and not by incentive for cures. Sociopaths which include politicians are drawn to places of power and money. Washington, London and Ottawa are typical centers where policy on health care is established by these sociopaths appearing to care, and political lobbyists and special interest groups are swarming with billions of dollars in bribe money and "special gifts" to get their way. This system perpetuates the cycle of corruption. Do you think that Bills before the Senate and Congress, written by the pharmaceuticals and health care providers are in the interest of the people? Maybe it's time to rethink how the system isn't working?

The trouble of changing a system that works for profit and not the people it serves, is that the vested interests controlling the system have no incentive for change. "Change" was the theme of President Obama's campaign. We just saw more of the same. Profit has no incentive to change since profit is working well for the individuals that currently control the system.

Your back pain will require surgery.
You will need to take these pills for the rest of your life.
The behavior of your child requires medication.
But who is telling the doctors what to say?

The current health care system treats the symptom instead of the cause

The healthcare system operates under a monopoly that trains doctors to assume the patient is properly nourished, toxic free, hormone balanced and living in a stress-free environment and autoimmune free. This is the point at which essential information is omitted from the doctor's training and where the system departs from practicing healthcare. The current system in place is trauma-care trained doctors practicing health care and the symptom is "sick care". Patients are presenting themselves to their doctors for treatment but are having the underlying causes of obesity, illness, and disease ignored in favor of playing with symptoms. You shouldn't consider using sick care other than for diagnosis, trauma care, birth and death, or you face getting on their treadmill of "sick care" having only your symptoms treated. All you have to do is believe that there might be a better way.

It is the power of authority absent of common sense that is suppressing the flow of information of doctors who write about cures or solutions to disease. Authority isn't pursuing a cure for anything otherwise they statistically would have found cures. I found that cures to health problems are no more difficult than giving your truck a tune up, cleaning some filters, and choosing a clean high octane fuel for it to run on to blow out some of the carbon build up. Doctors are trained to "conform" to a system of belief that is rigid where genius is suppressed. Collectively, society is operating in a system of belief, hopelessly immersed in ego and not on a system of truth with tragic results.

Cures are not allowed to be talked about in any part of health care but I should clear the air about my definition of what a cure is. If an MS patient goes in for a stint operation using a walker aid, and jumps off the table following an outpatient procedure and is walking his dog that night, to me that is a cure. So a cure by my definition is a profound improvement with an ailment. Is there anyone who disagrees? The only discussion that the current health care system talks about are recognizing and treating symptoms. This is a recipe for failure that is having successful results for everyone but the patient.

I wasted 36 years of my life going from one doctor to another until I was forced to free myself on my own from a wheelchair with cancer. Over that time I learned about real "health care". No health discipline was "wrong", but there is no health discipline that is "right". Combining the disciplines to achieve true health is in this book that was provided to me by hundreds of different doctors and people like myself with ideas. Collectively, we came to solve the Matrix pyramid and the sequence to obesity and disease for all. We could reduce health to 5 basic essential elements. The pyramid is the fulcrum of 5 elements from where the sequence of disease and obesity begins. By understanding the sequence to disease you understand how to reverse disease. By reversing it earlier in the sequence at the point where imbalances occur, you avoid, pain, inflammation, medication, scar tissue, disease, cancer, missed time at work, and accelerate healing to a point of thriving. Thriving is about realizing potential and precious few achieve this status.

The pyramid of health works for every ailment that gets in the way of a person thriving and reaching potential. The goal of the book is for everyone to find their potential of someone who is 10 years younger. My hope is that the statement will intrigue people to read on to find what I believe is the truth to curing yourself. It worked for me and 100's of others 100% who put in 100% effort. I realize I am not allowed to cure anyone but from using information put forth in the book, you can! Everyone who did, thrived.

I cured myself of:

- Cancer from a wheel chair where chemo didn't work, yet the cancer clinic counts me as their success. Statistics and assumptions can be misleading.
- Autoimmune disease gone, and proven 100% on 10,000 patients.
- Chronic Fatigue after enduring 36 years, gone.
- Osteoporosis so bad I broke my femur twice while walking. My bones are now that of someone 20 years younger than my peers confirmed by a bone scan, gone.
- Asthma completely gone.
- Allergies after enduring 36 years, gone.
- A pot belly, gone.
- A chronic headache I had for 36 years 24/7 hours a day and in occasionally in physical agony, gone.
- I'm now rollerblading for miles and bench pressing 150% of my weight.

Perhaps people should have a right to choice despite what authority allows. After my experience, the path provided by the health care system is not a choice I would follow.

Disease is the absence of health

An alkaline diet or a phytonutrient (plant based nutrient) diet gets your blood alkaline. My conclusions are that blood only becomes alkaline pH 7.0(+/- 0.2) being absent of inflammation, to sustain life and vitality to your cells. PH is the report card of the 5 elements that make up the Matrix pyramid of patient health. The blood's delivery of an abundance of high density nutrients to the cells, and the blood's ability to efficiently remove toxins makes up the equation to determine pH and the existence of inflammation.

Summary Points of Symptom:

Other than trauma, inflammation is caused by 1 or more of the 5 elements of health out of balance, everything else is just a symptom, and therefore the following can be cured by correcting the imbalances:

- To cure pain, know that pain is a symptom of inflammation.
- To cure disease, know that disease is a symptom of inflammation over time.
- To cure cancer, know that cancer is a symptom of inflammation over a longer period of time.
- To cure obesity, know that obesity is a symptom of inflammation.

Time is of the Essence

INFLAMMATION is the precursor to disease that leads to cancer with or without pain. Inflammation can significantly affect your energy levels. Pain, Disease, and Cancer naturally happens when inflammation is persistent over time and it results in the break down of cells and cellular chemistry, as they relate to one another in the body.

PAIN is a signaler, it is how your body talks to you and its best you don't ignore the symptoms of what your body is telling you. Pain means stop what you are doing, stop using what is sore. It means now. Being absent of pain will leave your cells in tact absent of cellular degeneration and permanent scarring.

OBESITY is a symptom of inflammation and not a symptom of eating too much or about counting calories, or lack of exercise, those are just symptoms and not the cause. Obesity is not a disease as the FDA is alleging, but a symptom of "5 elements out of balance" which results in obesity, a symptom of inflammation. Treating symptoms of obesity only leads to more obesity. Treating symptoms intensifies problems because it ignores the factor of time as it relates to cellular degeneration in the sequence that leads to disease.

Solving Health, is about Imbalance(s) and not the Symptom

The difference between being in a hospital bed, existing behind a walker, or living day to day in a traffic jam with a sore back to thriving, can be manipulated by the 5 elements of the Matrix for anyone. Pain, inflammation, obesity, medication, and the future of elective surgery are a thing of the past and simply a choice of whether you want to follow your doctor for more of the same, or follow the steps in the book. None of us knows what there still is to know, but here is information that can give us access to the ladder of life on how to thrive now. My hope is to tap into the potential energy of the healthy individual, where change of the system will come about as a result.

I've learned so much from my mistakes... I'm thinking of making a few more.

Chapter 1

The Matrix And the Sequence to Obesity and Disease

What is wrong with you is the mirror image of what is right with you. To thrive to the point where you can throw away your walker and get back to hiking, you need to be absent of inflammation and the word "can't". It's easy to get rid of disease and obesity and it's done by embracing health. Ultimate health is ultimate potential and to achieve it you need to practice a few equations.

Health is the least understood science on the planet and is the most important. You are not going to get to where you want to go unless you understand how to get there. Curing disease is about focusing on health. There are only 5 elements to health, "what your body needs and doesn't need". The body doesn't waste anything and operates at 100% efficiency even in a state of deficiency. No one or anything knows more about health than your body. The body came from a single cell to grow a heart, a brain, blood, skin, eyes. 50+ trillion cells that began from a single cell from a mother's womb who supplied nourishment absent of toxins. You can't reverse engineer nature as you are led to believe. We know what those cells need to achieve ultimate health. Today there are more than 200 chemicals in a newborn's umbilical cord and more than 75,000 chemicals developed since WW2 that are in the food chain along with that came autism and ADHD. Chemicals are toxins that are not only life sustaining but when combined are deadly to your body and your body's reaction to chemicals and malnutrition is inflammation that manifest negatively both physically, mentally and energetically. They are easy to recognize on the sides of your food packaging as words you have never heard before. "Natural or fresh" are common words that mean "put package back on shelf and run". Inflammation over time damages cells and leads to scar tissue. The goal is not only to eliminate inflammation but to accelerate the recovery. Little knowledge of anatomy is required to achieve optimum health and eliminate any disease, and it's so easy to do. All you need is time and a road map. Belief has no business interfering with 50+ trillion cells that have an ability to run at 100% efficiency while under deficiency. The body can run at 100% efficiency even when you are thirsty, hungry, hot, tired, toxic or malnourished.

One observation I made, was if you reduce acute inflammation in one area by 50%, you will improve overall condition of the entire body by 50% by every measure there is. Health is like the water in your aquarium. When the level falls you expose the rocks of past traumas and gene weakness called "disease". Resolution of disease only happens when the water level of health in your aquarium rises and the symptoms of disease submerge. This is the definition of "cure", or what doctors refer to as remission. Remission means that "the rocks are still there submerged for potential problems to re-emerge in the future, if you allow your level of health to fall".

With trauma, pain comes first and then inflammation. This type of inflammation is the current expertise of the present system of trauma care practicing health care.

With disease inflammation comes first, then pain and or weight gain. This is where the current system of health care fails miserably.

Anyone who dies of natural causes will die brought on by a nutritional deficiency, perhaps compounded by toxicity issues, hormone(s) deficiency, and autoimmune symptoms for which the cure has been found.

Disease caused by nutritional deficiency was proven with Scurvy as a vitamin C deficiency, Muscular Dystrophy is a selenium deficiency, congestive heart failure is brought on by primarily by one deficiency of B1 thiamine. Most infertility is because of low iodine. Nutrient loading of 77 minerals you can find in Nevada helps. Most ADD and ADHD can be rid of with meal replacement containing those 77 minerals, 16 vitamins, 3 EFA's, 18 amino acids, along with avoidance of sugar, GMO, gluten, vaccination and the child or patient is living mold free. It helps make the drug Ritalin irrelevant. It has been proven that 83% of breast cancer is caused by low iodine, and the other 17% is responsible by contamination of xenoestrogens. Other than radiation, most diseases begin with a combination of low nutrients and contamination of the body with toxins found in almost all food and products sold in a grocery store. Autoimmune is different (see chapter 3)

The cure for everything is the same. It's about what your body needs and eliminating what it doesn't, (see chapter 2). Edema, hair loss, hypothyroidism, cold hands and feet, bone or breast cancer, is an iodine deficiency, and with cancer you add oxygen to your regiment of healing. With colon cancer you should add aloe vera gel in a glass of water while you are doing oxygen treatment to repair the digestive tract more effectively than any hospital can offer you.

My question is, why not everyone take all the 114 nutrients in one meal replacement, an extra iodine supplement, and do some juicing of organic vegetables and fruit and be awesome? As you go through life, the belief of the population is to drink more tap water and shop for the best price in a grocery store. Both will kill you slowly as your health descends into a medicine cabinet to keep you alive. I bet that any millionaire would prefer to give up his wealth and trade that to walk a beach and be free from a wheelchair. I did.

Oxygen stops disease when health fails:

For all those who are in fear, know that all disease is anaerobic and oxygen is aerobic. Dosed properly, oxygen can kill the flower of disease within 30 days for less than 1$. But you must change the soil in which the flower of disease grew. Oxygen will take out the disease, but will not correct the cause of inflammation and pain that lead to cancer. Oxygen is great to use when time is of the essence. Diseased cells and cancer can only exist in a body that lacks oxygen and those cells thrive off sugar. Sugar renders white blood cells useless within 20 minutes.

Oxygen kills virus and or bacteria that are responsible for the diseases of AIDS, HIV, hepatitis, pneumonia, and flesh eating disease. Oxygen destroys what doesn't belong in the body and makes the use of vaccinations obsolete. It has excellent results for IBS because it takes out anaerobic cells (candida) that cause IBS, but your tolerance of concentration is difficult to get absolute results. Taking the equivalent of 40 drops of oxygen buffered in an aloe solution is the best proprietary idea I have heard of to have intense effect on cancer, IBS and disease like AIDS. Oxygen is like a healing bomb to a diseased body and works as fast as you can tolerate the toxicity of cell die-off, called Herxheimer's effect. The doctor who found the cure for autoimmune also found the solution to Herxheimer's with a special diet and a "pre-treatment" prescription for 10 days that most Lyme patients and treating physicians would like to hear about (see chapter 3). Taking oxygen is far superior to antibiotics and less expensive, but you need direction and patience.

Oxygen will not work for the disease of autoimmune or MS that come from exposure to neurotoxins but can help eliminate inflammation to take out those diseased cells that result from it. Oxygen can only be taken temporarily for 3-4 weeks maximum in concentration because it is a little caustic. There is a stabilized form of oxygen (11% ozone) you can take daily with food that will lower inflammation in your body to prevent disease, sold at a health food store. Who thought that the health food store could promote health?

Oxygen works by the free oxygen molecule sourced from either h2o2 (hydrogen peroxide food grade), ozone (o3), and chlorine dioxide (clo2) sold as MMS (miracle mineral supplement), with all methods oxidizing anaerobic cells. All 3 must be ramped up gently because of Herxheimer's effect, perhaps a drop or 2/day, increase a drop per day as you can tolerate to be safe. You have to be cautious taking oxygen because the die off of dead diseased cells turn toxic through the elimination process and are reabsorbed back into the blood in the colon. Watch for signs of headaches, and nausea to know you aren't drinking enough water to flush. At maximum dose, expect disease to be eliminated within 30 days. Using hyperbaric chambers for the absorption of oxygen under pressure, can be a more gentle method to take. Cardio is good for preventing inflammation because oxygen exchange in the capillaries of the lungs becomes efficient at enriching the blood with oxygen and keeping your cells healthy.

Oxygen works so well that there are cases in Canada where a cancer patient has had less than a month to live and was brought back to full recovery with oxygen along with nutrition, supplements and cleansing. I proved this for someone in his 90's sent home by 6 oncologists who only had 60 days to live with cancer in his lungs, liver, stomach and digestive tract (colon). With only a week of this treatment, he went from being carried into the house, to walking to the store 90 days later with only 1 week of treatment. His "palliative care" team were perplexed and have stopped calling. There are 2 things that must be done to cure disease, one is to kill the flower of disease and the other is to change your soil that led to disease in the first place. Without correcting the imbalances, the flower of disease almost always comes back.

Correcting your imbalances corrects your soil to a healthy alkaline 7.0pH (-+.02). Cancer is just a symptom of inflammation over time. Soil is the blood of your body, like oil is to your engine, like water is the blood of the earth. To keep disease and cancer out of your body you need to improve your soil and the condition of it through manipulating the 5 elements (because this is so foreign a thought, it is worth repeating).

Oxygen makes chlorine, bromine and fluoride, irrelevant in your drinking water, pools and hot tubs. All 3 are approaching toxicity levels of arsenic and all 3 are absorbed in the body and are cumulative and not surprising, are responsible and contribute to a whole host of diseases that many charities claim to be trying to conquer, including obesity.

Note: you must follow instructions before you take oxygen h2o2 food grade. Oxygen is great if you are in a hurry, and it is also an effective tool to kill anaerobic cells, working like a parachute to help where time is of the essence. Oxygen is friendly to life and unfriendly to diseased cells that don't belong in your body, unlike chemo which is just unfriendly. MMS is effective at targeting diseased cells and leaving healthy cells intact and h2o2 (food grade from a health food store) is the cheapest.

Treating 100 patients of cancer with h2o2 food grade is about $100 and treating 100 people with chemo costs about $10 million. The benefit of taking oxygen, is that as you take it to cure disease you become healthier and the survival rate is close to 100%. As you take chemo you get sicker and weaker and the survival rate is close to 0%. With oxygen therapy you can keep working and with chemo you can't. Chemo is a very toxic chemical and the nurses that dispense it must wear rubber gloves.

Health

To evolve as a species, chemicals must be removed from the food chain where they find their way into your body and begin the cycle of inflammation and disease. We can't afford to remain sick, dumbed down in brain fog absent of Life Force energy to live. As long as you're healthy, money will look after itself. You can't do it from a hospital bed.

When you have pain and inflammation in your body and/or you are obese over a period of time, you are halfway to developing cancer, or you are halfway to thriving. Health care has a monopoly and makes and enforces its own laws. When you arrive at their doors they assess you and assume that you are nourished absent of toxins. But that is the underlying purpose of your visit when Life Force energy has left your body and has been replaced with disease. Asking your doctor to help cure your disease is like taking your car that needs a tune up to an auto body mechanic. Both are skilled but you are asking the wrong mechanic for help.

Your body's ability to heal is greater than anyone has permitted you to believe

To simplify how easy it is to cure yourself of disease, you should look at your body like you would your car. The regular maintenance you do on your car is to change the oil, the filters, be sure to put clean gasoline in the tank, and blow out some carbon. Love is the air in your tires and rust is the inflammation. How does this compare to what you are doing for your body? Your gasoline is your food for your body. Make sure your food is clear of toxins and as natural to the earth and alive as possible, and high octane organic is best. The Life Force energy of your food choices acts like the cooling system of your car engine, cooling the flames of inflammation. The filters are for eliminating toxins and waste that don't belong but you must clean them once in a while and there is more than one (see Chapter 6).

THE HEALTH MATRIX

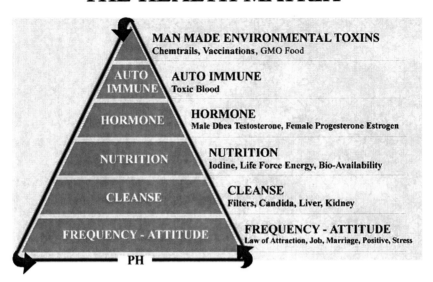

The 5 Elements
Affecting pH/ Inflammation/ Pain/ Disease/ Cancer/ Obesity/ Immunity/ Dementia/ Potential

TOXIC BLOOD (autoimmune) is at the top of the pyramid of health and the most important element that negatively affects pH. Toxic blood has the biggest negative impact on the elements below it in the Matrix. The medical community has not connected the cause of autoimmune disease to exposure to toxic mold yet but science has. If neurotoxins from exposure to toxic mold are present in the blood, the cytokine response will destroy hormones and even if you are on a healthy diet for the right blood type, autoimmune will simply destroy every system that is in its path including the immune system, and cause depression proportionately to the level of neurotoxins in your blood over time. It is caused from living, working, or vacationing in a moldy environment. The body's inability to repair itself is a key problem of patients with this source of inflammation who have symptoms of autoimmune.

Most don't know when they are being exposed and 24% of patients will have the dreaded DNA type measured on chromosome 6 of the innate immune system that will leave you unable to excrete neurotoxins even after you have removed yourself from a toxic moldy environment. This is contrary to the doctor's handbook of practice. The 24% of patients with this gene-type will go on to experience autoimmune disease over time in relation to the intensity of the infestation even after removing themselves from mold. 76% are not susceptible to permanent symptoms and will cough it off within days and weeks following exposure after leaving a moldy environment because they have the gene-type that allow the neurotoxins to be excreted out the digestive tract. But 100% of every patient that lives in mold will experience chronic fatigue and symptoms of autoimmune. I believe that mononucleosis is autoimmune misdiagnosed from being in a moldy environment. My theory for mono could be proven by a basic blood test found in the autoimmune chapter (3). There are only a handful of doctors that know how to diagnose and treat autoimmune disease, but don't get too excited, because they are not permitted to treat patients by the regulatory boards having authority. Authority can be very dangerous.

2. HORMONES are the 2nd most important element below Toxic blood on the pyramid that affects pH. Balanced healthy levels of hormones allow for poor diets, nutritional deficiencies, toxic livers and kidneys, stressful environments, and people will still have a relatively healthy pH and plentiful energy, absent of mold. The aging process begins when cellular death exceeds the rate of cellular rejuvenation and is accelerated as hormones fall. Bioidentical hormones are the most effective method of slowing the aging process virtually making cosmetic surgery, creams, botox, medication, loss of collagen, and diseases associated with old age irrelevant. This is the element when lacking that has the most impact on aging and osteoporosis.

3. NUTRITION is the 3rd most important element to affect pH and inflammation I call the gasoline of your car without the sugar in the tank. Blood that is free of neurotoxins and rich with bio-available hormones, is the point where nutrition comes in as number 3 on the list of most important elements that affect health, the measure of pH, and super immunity. There are some key principles borrowed from the science of

fractality that best explains its importance. Nutrition is a big subject I made small, by juicing, eating organic fruits and vegetables as well as meal replacements with 114 essential nutrients contained that got me out of my wheelchair with no exercising in 2 weeks after being atrophied for close to 2 years. Meal replacement is like a health food store in a canister, so doing this diet is all I had to learn about nutrition other than supplements. You cannot get all your nutrients from the 4 food groups as the health care industry suggests. Organic only maintains health, and doesn't accelerate recovery. For non-organic products and food, your body will deteriorate and age faster. With fast food deterioration is at an acclerated rate.

4. TOXIC TISSUE is the 4th most important element that affects pH. It is the health of your organs, I call your filters that are significant for recovery that get you up a few levels of health that are key to thriving. Your filters need to be absent of toxins and inflammation, and it is primarily the liver, and secondary the digestive tract, and third the kidneys. Sweating through your skin, and even your breathing allows for the excretion of toxins from your body. I will list some cleanses that will boost your pH, increase your nutrient absorption, lower inflammation throughout your body to reduce chronic headaches, aches, pain, and excess weight and boost immunity. Even IQ can be boosted, reducing brain fog all by cleansing. The 3.5lb/1.5kg liver is a filter that takes a lot of work to clear but is essential to thrive. I know people who got off kidney dialysis by cleansing their kidneys and livers of toxins and "stones". Imagine how that improved their vitality. A toxic liver is a major cause of hypertension and weight gain.

5. FREQUENCY refers to your vitality or vibration of your mood as it pertains to your Life Force energy. If you live in a toxic free environment that is stress free, conducive to you following your passion or bliss without shame or guilt, it will have a positive affect and can raise your pH over time. Love is the highest vibration for raising your pH. If you are in love with someone or something, with the other elements in balance, stress will roll off your shoulders. With euphoric energy high and stress-draining energy low, you could find yourself walking, running, exercising more often to blow off excess energy after a day's work. Finding opportunities and having more luck are common. If you are getting arrested in a drug bust with

guns pointed at your head your pH could fall quickly but that drop in pH won't be supported by your overall health of your cells. So a rebound will be quick once you get over the shock, have processed and accepted your situation. It's how you cope with stress that matters. The people who laugh it off thrive and the people who brood will have trouble by embracing poor health habits and circles of friends that support negativity.

Toxic habits seem to co-exist in toxic environments. Misery loves company. Bad or unhealthy habits can pull you into a vortex that has a spiraling affect that can pull you down. In a situation where you lose your lover, your job, or your house is going into foreclosure and stress is over a prolonged period of time, pH drop can make you sick if you can't find a release mechanism like luck or laughter.

Pathetic is temporary and you can be thankful for the lessons you learn from it. Perhaps you can go to the beach and pitch a tent, tell the foreclosure manager at the bank you need your minivan for a while longer? Laughing helps.

The interesting opinion of people is they associate medicine as if they are vitamins. Yes they can be helpful, but medicine is only meant to be taken temporarily to suspend symptoms until a cause can be corrected. Long term use of medicine should only be for perhaps 1% of the population, but currently that statistic is 70% in North America, and that doesn't include over the counter drugs. Inflammation is like rust is to steel over time. Wheelchairs shouldn't be the motivator to you trying to achieve your potential, but perhaps falling in love with something or someone should.

MAN MADE TOXINS may be the new king to the top of the Matrix pyramid that destroys health for North Americans. Vaccinations, GMO and chemtrails are having devastating effects on health that may trump the 170 diseases of autoimmune combined. They have been introduced in the last 20 years, but their toxicity levels and intensity has been ramped up in the last couple of years.

pH

The measure of the 5 elements of the Health Matrix is pH. It is a function of your inflammation and thus a measure of your health. Your ability to deal with stress is directly related with pH. People who have alkaline pH deal with stress gracefully and effortlessly. Optimum health is measured at an optimum blood level of 7.0 (+/-0.2) pH. Inflammation begins below 6.8 and disease begins below a pH of 6.2. Cancer begins at a blood level below 5.6 pH and below 5.0 pH in time, you will be dead. 5.0 pH is 100 times more acidic than 7.0 pH and the symptom interferes with nutrient absorption. At 7.0 pH, you are either thriving or you will be thriving. It is interesting to note that Osteoporosis, a common problem among the +50 crowd and especially in women is caused by acidic pH of the blood, a symptom of high inflammation over time. Osteoporosis is just a symptom. It is best to determine between "symptom and cause". That is the compass of your roadmap to recovery.

Bioavailability and Life Force energy, the nutrient density of what you eat helps move your pH up. The less waste and the more Life Force your food has, the less work your body will have integrating into its cells for energy and repair. The higher the absorption rate and the less waste your body has to expend for removal, the better for lowering inflammation. Better means that your blood will go alkaline to 7.0pH along with super immunity, increased IQ and energy. Your IQ, energy levels, and motivation correlate to inflammation.

Note: you can drop dead with a healthy pH with no signs of inflammation if you are for example a runner. By taxing nutrients intensely on a broad spectrum running and not replacing according to a broad spectrum of deficiencies over time can drop the high school basketball player or long distance runner with perfect cholesterol levels dead.

Measuring pH

Measuring pH by saliva/urine test paper measures your diet pH which can fluctuate drastically throughout the day with the consumption of Vega meal replacement or Chlorella/ Spirulina that are alkaline in nature. The saliva/ urine pH fluctuates like a car's tachometer. In first gear the tachometer can move quickly with your diet but not with the speed reflected as a measure of your blood pH. Moving the blood pH takes months to see results and weeks if you use methods that accelerate the correction of imbalances at "turbo charge" recovery. PH is a very little understood measure of health because the solutions have been elusive on how to achieve optimum pH by any opinion I have heard or read. So when I had cancer my blood pH was 5.0, and my daily pH paper tests fluctuated over 8.0 depending on what I was eating day to day and throughout the day and could be influenced by the pH of my food from the previous day. It is best to wait a minimum of 12 hours and 24 hours is better to get more accurate results from pH paper testing. And where do you get pH paper, a health food store of course.

PH is the measure of super immunity, a function of hydrogen and an indication of the highest level of health there is. Organic lemons and limes can move your blood to alkaline. But non organic lemons and limes can bring your pH down theoretically based on an 80-90% reduction in nutrients associated with "growing life with poisonous pesticides" as an ingredient in the soil. Despite what people think, pesticides main detriment to disease and acidifying pH tests lies in the fact that they kill the organisms in the ground that transfer Life Force nutrients from the soil to the plant by up to 90%. I think alkaline diets are emphasized because they are typical of healthy live vegetarian fare. Healthy food tends to be alkaline but it is not the alkalinity of it that moves your blood pH up. If you focus on vegetables and fruits that are alkaline and miss out on the concept of diversity that will actually contribute to acidification of your blood, the opposite of desired results.

A way to measure inflammation is by using the sediment rate blood test that focuses on inflammation and blood proteins. If you have inflammation in your body then dead cells are released from the site of inflammation as cellular death that then circulate in the bloodstream as a protein. The erythrocyte sedimentation rate (ESR), C-reactive protein (CRP) and plasma viscosity (PV) blood tests are commonly used to detect this increase in protein and are the markers of inflammation. There are other ways to measure inflammation of abnormal blood levels that are the cause of inflammation. The blood tests for autoimmune are available in the US but not in Canada. Health care treats the cause of inflammation and trauma care treats the symptoms, both are great providing the patient gets the appropriate care for the condition presented.

There are 12 sources of Inflammation that cause disease and suggested remedy
(Malnutrition and autoimmune lead to arthritis compounded by the other 10)

Natural sources of Inflammation (including cancer) that can be "reduced" by oxygen:

1. Toxic blood from Biotoxin source, called Auto immune disease.

   Remedy: change building code and pull occupancy permits on moldy units that make people sick.

2. Nutrition can be corrected by spiking nutrient density and diversity.

   Remedy: Eliminate toxins from food and eliminate nutrient damaging food handling & processing like pasteurization.

3. Toxic liver and tissue corrected by flushing then cleansing the liver.

   Remedy: incentives to those who flush and clean their livers.

4. Hormones can be corrected and optimized with bioidentical hormones.

   Remedy: Everyone get hormones balanced after age 40 and checked periodically before 40 by blood test.

5. Stress you can either embrace stress or let it go as a lesson and laugh at life.

   Remedy: More recreation, reduced bills, better health.

Natural sources of Inflammation that can be "eliminated" by oxygen:

6. Virus
7. Bacteria

The susceptibility of these 2 increase as pH and immunity falls.

Remedy by oxygen. Boron is effective but expensive, h2o2 hydrogen peroxide food grade is cheap and effective but difficult to take, MMS is effective and price effective, hyperbaric chamber is easy and helps, h2o2 can be effective by intravenous, oxygen with aloe vera is most effective.

Man Made sources of Inflammation we can avoid and need to stop:

8. Radiation we need to avoid in our world of paranoia.
9. GMO's are in 80% of our food that is non-organic. Avoidance is the only remedy.
10. Vaccinations, 100% of those vaccinated have some degree of autism as a consequence. PCA, chlorella, and chelation help get this deadly cocktail of toxins out of your blood.
11. Chemtrails are spraying harmful barium, strontium, radiation along with aluminum and a host of toxic chemicals criss-crossing our blue skies. Taking Bentonite clay from a health food store daily helps bind with those toxins to give relief. Morgellons disease is a consequence of man-made GMO's and chemtrails. Vaccinations are suspected but not confirmed. See chapter 8 for Morgellons. Morgellons should be renamed the "GMO disease."
12. Stress that is man-made are ambulance, police, fire truck sirens. Bull horns from trains that disturb life all hours of the night, harassment from police, revenue services, traffic jams that are engineered (they don't "just happen"), signs, conformity, authority, debt, poison in food and water, nutrients taken out of food, licenses for everything, destroy our sanctuary of peace in our communities.

Remedy: Change the governments where these happen.

Source of Inflammation we can't avoid:

Trauma, recovery can be cut in less than half the time by a patient with a clean liver and nutrient stores in the body filled. Patients with toxic livers, who are malnourished have trouble recovering from surgery and have problems with infection before, during and after.

Note: hospital trays are full of inflammatory food absent of nutrition and full of toxins.

Remedy: Less accidents will happen when: there are less toxins in the body, less stress, hormones balanced, quality nutrients feeding brain and central nervous system. Recovery times cut in half and more can be realized with change and adoption of basic principals.

Osteoporosis caused by acidic pH

Osteoporosis is the king of inflammation and you can point to a calendar when it is gone. 30 days is how long it takes to completly change the chemistry in your body. With osteoporosis, change of bone mass improves weeks and months to follow. Cancer is the king of inflammation gone wrong over a long period of time. For cancer complete chemistry of the body is only 2-4 weeks to eliminate the condition of cancer. There is virtually the same remedy for virtually every disease, one or 2 products different.

Autoimmune accelerates the decline of health faster and more absolute than all others Health Matrix elements combined. You need to consider this possibility or dismiss it before you move down the pyramid on your path to recovery. Autoimmune, MS, Chronic Lyme, obesity, mental illness and more involved.

Osteoporosis is not a disease but a condition created by acidic blood from a body that has overall inflammation and cellular degeneration over a period of time. The disease is a classic example of what happens when several elements go out of balance. Autoimmune is often a participant but not by itself, and because it is age related, it is hormone related. Its remedy is an example of how to cure disease and just about any disease by correcting imbalances, and calcium isn't one of them. That is just a symptom. Often bioidentical hormones is enough to correct osteoporosis.

As with all disease the "sequence" involves looking at eliminating autoimmune as the first suspect, 2nd reestablishing bioavailable hormones, 3rd spiking your nutrients with meal replacements, juicing organic fruit and vegetables and eliminate toxins from your food, 4th flushing and cleansing your liver, kidneys and digestive tract of parasites and stones, and 5th find pleasure with the simple things in life. Absent of autoimmune concerns, bioidentical hormones will have the biggest effect at eliminating osteoporosis. Osteoporosis takes time to regenerate bone health integrity and it is not necessary doing all 5 elements. By doing all 5 not only accelerates recovery, and every health issue in your body but along with it some issues you didn't know you had because you got used to them. Patients actually get used to pain and low energy. I did and had no idea how much pain I was in until I was able to rapidly release it eliminating autoimmune disease from my body. Unless you experience trauma, decline in health is imperceptible but recovery can be rapid and dramatic when you correct the 5 imbalances at the same time.

Osteoporosis is easiest to overcome by taking bio identical hormones because it ranks #2 in the pyramid and access to this treatment is available off the internet cheaply or with precision by a bioidentical hormone specialist doctor MD. These doctors don't necessarily have any "extra" training but just an interest. Autoimmune is hardest to beat because access to treatment is almost impossible to get. If you have autoimmune, you will need to focus on the next 3 until the health care system catches up to ethics or people demand it from their doctor and the system. It will take changing the whole system. There is a long road ahead, but every obstacle overcome leads to a better tomorrow. We just have to refuse to take "no" for an answer. The cure for autoimmune and every disease has been found. Best to follow the dos and don'ts in chapter 2 and the other chapters as a guide to eliminate inflammation.

People overestimate their health and underestimate their disease

Application of the Matrix

To evaluate yourself make a list that differentiates the cause from the symptoms of inflammation of your disease.

Someone who asked me for help had:

Diabetes, rheumatoid arthritis (RA), osteoporosis, depression, edema, cold hands and an inflamed liver. When I met him I asked, "where are you getting the mold from?" Mold is the cause of his rheumatoid arthritis, and most everything else are just symptoms of the RA and low iodine. Disease comes from the top down. The source of mold turned out to be in his bedroom and he needed to repaint the walls each spring because they would become discolored over the winter from mold behind the walls.

The mold created the symptoms in his body as pain in his neck, back, hands, knees, and feet that caused chronic fatigue along with headaches, poor sleep, depression, and lethargy. The autoimmune would be the primary cause of inflammation in the pancreas to give him diabetes along with gallstones from bilary sludge from being chronically sick and malaise with a poor diet.

His stomach was bloated because of an inflamed liver from the toxic mountain of medication he was on to deal with autoimmune, depression, osteoporosis, sleeplessness and diabetes. The other layer of fat around his middle was from having raised leptin levels caused by autoimmune and eating a regular diet of food absent of nutrition loaded with toxins. The other layer of fat was caused by low male hormones damaged from autoimmune and his age (51). The gallstones were still another layer of fat. Long term illness causes biliary sludge in the gallbladder and because he showered and drank in municipal tap water, that bleached out iodine to slow metabolism. The leptin hormone is a problem with autoimmune patients that causes fat cells to collect around the abdomen.

It didn't matter what I said or showed him, he was stuck so far down the rabbit hole of belief and fear under his doctor's care. His solution was to keep doing what he was doing and seek the advice of a nutritionist. The solution is to go through the pyramid of health starting with autoimmune, then spike the body with juicing and high density nutrients to rejuvenate inflamed cells, flush and then cleanse the liver, take extra iodine to eliminate edema and cold hands, and then follow with hormone replacement. But first you have to eliminate the mold. Autoimmune takes expertise to tackle with tests necessary, and is going to take a lot of demand to get it recognized. The protocol is the exact same protocol for osteoporosis.

Another example was of an elderly man in his mid-70's who had trouble walking to the end of his driveway. He didn't have any evidence of mold in his place nor symptoms of autoimmune. His doctor had diagnosed him with arthritis in his hips and bursitis in his shoulder. Living without his passion for hiking and legs failing him he told me he had no reason to live. His hips had failed less than a year ago, so scar tissue wasn't too much of a concern. To fix his hips and bursitis I needed to first take the pain out of his shoulder, knowing that good "rem" sleep is essential to recovery. With accupressure massaged into areas to the sympathetic muscles around his shoulder without disturbing the area in pain, I starved the blood to those that were in spasm which allowed for their release. Pressing on the muscle and holding for just over 30 seconds is long enough. With all significant areas pressed the pain was gone in the shoulder without touching the muscle in spasm after 30 minutes. The pain had been interfering with his sleep, and sleep is essential for prevention and recovery of any illness/inflammation throughout the whole body.

With immediate success I could coax more details. His hips gave out over the last 6 months and the bursitis came about as a fall on the concrete and his body's inability to repair itself. Bursitis is caused by malnutrition and was the major flag that was causing problems in his hips. We know that there are only 2 sources of inflammation for muscles. Autoimmune was ruled out so nutrient deficiency was the problem. As you get old the problem of malnutrition is common because deficiency is cumulative. The remedy for him was about getting nutrition to the inflamed muscles in a hurry. Flushing toxins was the other objective. The more diverse and the higher the nutrient density, the faster the recovery. Muscle pain and arthritis are a symptom of nutrient deficiency so a plan with iodine, chlorella, a liver flush, a couple of liver cleanses, and a pail of high density meal replacement containing minerals, vitamins, proteins and 18 amino acids 2x/day until the canister was finished was what he could afford on a fixed income. He was hiking up a mountain 8 miles on the 16th day without pain almost 2 years ago. The interesting thing with him and everyone in a state of nutrient deficiency, is that up to the day before profound relief is felt there are no improvements. Improvement is profound and immediate for everyone. On the 15th day he remained invalid. The 16th day he experienced euphoria.

Another example in his late 80's took an hour to get out of bed with painful spasms running through his legs each morning. One week on the high density nutrient was all it took to clear up that problem and it hasn't returned in a couple of years. Again profound improvement was on the 7th day and the pain was gone. Up to day 6, he remained invalid. He went back to playing hour long doubles tennis without taking a break on the 8th day.

Another example in her mid-50's diagnosed with arthritis in her hips was unable to get up the stairs one step at a time upright or into bed because the pain was so bad. The arthritis had escalated for over a year and hip replacement was going to be necessary soon according to her doctor. Within 2 weeks on the meal replacement the pain was gone and for over 2 ½ years, function is completely back to normal even though she drinks a case of soda a week, smokes, enjoys alcohol and drinks coffee every morning all of which interferes with nutrient absorption. Her nutrient deficiency was cumulative and maintenance is minimal when using the superior Life Force energy of meal replacement in a glass of water once a day from a health food store. The meal replacement in pharmacies and regular grocery stores have a life force energy like that of a twinkie…well almost, because they contain so many sources of GMO's that put your body into inflammation contributing to IBS disease even though their marketing promotes itself as the answer to health and nutrition. People are buying the hoax by the case from grocery stores, being recommended by doctors and handed out to patients in hospitals as the answer to malnutrition. The product's attributes are misleading to point of being criminal, and there is more than one type of these products on the market.

Another example had irritable bowel syndrome. He had a hard time walking from the pain in his lower stomach, which is common today because of GMO's are in 80% of food sold in regular grocery stores. He took 20 drops of oxygen in a glass of water on an empty stomach and the next day was running! He had an iron belly to take 20 drops, so be careful to start with perhaps 3 drops and increase each day until you get to maximum dose as your gut will allow from the toxic die off. I found it best to do 2x/day and go from 3 drops in the morning and 6 drops in the evening and 10 drops the next morning and 15 drops that evening and try 20 drops the next morning and evening for a week or 2 and chase with quality probiotics for weeks and high quality organic food so as not to destroy your hard fought gut flora health. Headaches and nausea are a sign of herxheimer's that you need to cut back on your oxygen dose or increase drinking water to allow your body to rid itself of toxins from die off of anaerobic diseased cells gently. Drinking a lot of water to flush toxins out your body is a good idea an hour or so after taking oxygen. Try to stop coffee, alcohol, soda, television and microwaving permanently. You can find a lot of probiotics in organic sour krout if you are on a budget. Bread, milk, sugar, beer, alcohol, and red meat are bad for gut flora. You will handle stress better with a strong gut flora absent of IBS with improved energy.

Another example is someone who is a president of a multinational corporation, who had Wry disease or commonly called Torticollis of the neck. 10 days on high density nutrient meal replacement cleared it up permanently 2 years ago, even though his liver is plugged with gallstones and parasites. The nutrients got rid of the inflammation and his neck returned back to normal movement. He endured 1 year of pain before he asked me for help.

Another example was a farmer in his mid-50's who transformed his life in less than 3 weeks by taking the high density nutrition, probiotics, iodine, a glutathione supplement in a canister you can't buy in a store, and a liver cleanse. It turned back his biological clock 10 years and eliminated most of the pain in his legs he was experiencing from a hangover of Lou Gherig's disease. The relief was so profound he could go back to full days working on the farm with tremendous energy in only 3 weeks!

Another example who by medical terms is obese tried unsuccessfully for years at every weight loss clinic there was on TV and in the newspapers to lose weight and was scheduled to have half her stomach removed and was under observation for a liver transplant. She was on 500 calories a day and had an exercise bike but still couldn't lose a pound for years. She lost 26 lbs. in 30 days by just taking iodine and doing 4 liver cleanses from Isagenix.com. She could have tripled her daily calorie intake and could have lost 26 lbs. every month until she hit healthy weight, by reading the chapter on weight loss. The surgery for her stomach was cancelled and she was taken off the list as a candidate for liver transplant, 2 ½ years ago.

Joe was an individual in his 20's who got a job starting on an oil rig. He completed his first shift of a few weeks in northern Alberta and it nearly killed him. Muscles inflamed going hard all day on long back to back shifts, he didn't think his body could make another shift. He was motivated and wanted to buy a house but was on probation. I gave him a pail of high density meal replacement for the 2 weeks he was off before he began his next shift. By the end of his second shift he got removed from probation, placed full time and got promoted. He moved through his days with boundless energy and the cold no longer bothered him while he finished his second canister.

Alan was an individual who has skin psoriasis. He thought it was his liver and his thoughts that affected his problem. First off psoriasis is not a disease, but a symptom of a disease. It is caused by environmental mold or biotoxin exposure. To get rid of Psoriasis you need to get out of mold, the cause of psoriasis. To get rid of the symptom you need to remove neurotoxins from your blood with Olestyr (Cholestyramine) 2 grams 4x/day on an empty stomach for 15 days. To lower another symptom of abnormally high TNF-b1 levels take Larch tree extract, a natural nutritional supplement for 15$. The current medical protocol suggests removing your immune system at a cost of 1000's of dollars to lower TNF levels for autoimmune disease. The damage done with this course of treatment is devastating to your body, your bank account and to those whose finances won't allow treatment, a blessing in disguise.

I had a friend with an infection in her gallbladder and instead of flushing and cleaning it for a few hundred dollars over a handful of weekends, she chose to have it removed for free. She didn't know that this will shorten her quality of life by years, and she will have digestion problems trying to break down fats in her diet for the rest of her life. She had flirted with undiagnosed rheumatoid arthritis for years and inflammation makes your bile in your gallbladder become thick and over time gallstones further complicate inflammation. She is content to be on pain killers off and on for the rest of her life. Perhaps it's the easiest path for her? But she had to quit her job because of pain and discomfort performing normal duties. She chose to trust her doctor and the option offered by the system. When a gallbladder gets removed other organs aren't far behind.

I met a lady in her 60's who had Crohn's disease who was about to have part of her intestines cut out. I told her that 2 grams/4x/day on an empty stomach of Olestyr from her doctor for 2 weeks should do the trick and to be sure to stay away from mold. She only did half that amount 2x/ day for 2 weeks and the result was that she didn't need the surgery. She was happy and gave me a high five. It was one of her employees that told me about "sea salt" sold in regular grocery stores with 92% toxic content. My advice is to go organic only until we get some ethical standards from ethical politicians and that might be awhile.

Another man 57, didn't have the energy and couldn't get off the sofa for 1½ years despite dwindling finances and a mortgage with customers calling and wanting to do business. He didn't have the energy to return a phone call, he couldn't. He thought he was "burned out". Turns out he's on high blood pressure medication from years of drinking. Hyper tension can kill your energy. I got him on a couple of liver flushes followed by a couple of liver cleanses and some high density meal replacements along with probiotics, juicing and iodine. He went from the couch, to walking the dog, to jogging and working 60 hours a week looking forward to the next! He turned into a dynamo and was soon making some big money and back to handling a portfolio of customers within weeks. The funny thing about his story is that he never attributed success to cleaning, flushing the liver, or doing nutrients and supplements but recently doubled his order when he ran out.

As my own patient the remedy that worked for me to get me out of inflammation and my wheelchair was to first remove myself from mold. I then took CSM /Olestyr/ Chloestyramine Rx (same thing) 2 grams 4x/ day before meals and bed on an empty stomach in a glass of water and that lowered my pain substantially. I needed good gut flora (probiotics) to pass this mixture. It lowered the C3a and C4a blood tests that measure for inflammation over the 15 days I took it. The second step was to re-regulate abnormal blood levels. I took Cozaar Rx to reduce TGF-b1, called Transforming Growth Factor beta-1 for 10 days, which drastically reduced pain I didn't know I had. The last step for me and for most patients of autoimmune was to then take Vaso Intestinal Peptide (VIP) for several months to mitigate inflammation. VIP helps to restore low MSH (alpha melanocyte stimulating hormone), which increases endorphins, decreases sun burning, decreases sensitivity to pain, substantially lowers pain, and gives you a sense of well-being. There is a plethora of information on the topic of autoimmune simple step by step logic. But there are 10 different levels of treatment possible depending on HLA-dr, blood tests that display the DNA array on chromosome 6. There are 4 main solutions that can be drawn up in 5 minutes with a timeline to recovery for every patient diagnosed.

At commencement of the autoimmune treatment I had no legs to stand on, the muscle had withered away to the size of my ankles. The solution for me was taking Isagenix meal replacement which contain the equivalent of 10 meals in one glass of water. Within 2 weeks on this formula, I was able to stand up out of my wheelchair to a walker. It was my introduction to meal replacement that returned my atrophied legs back to normal after 2 weeks, and without physio or exercising. The third and final stage of treatment for autoimmune was VIP where my pain really went down. VIP was shipped on ice and taken 3 or 4 times a day sprayed up the nose. The VIP got me from a walker to crutches within a few weeks and then walking without crutches gingerly after a few months. I was rollerblading for miles within a year and I'm still doing so.

With cancer returning after chemo didn't work, was the biggest pain in my recovery. I learned later that chemo is a potent toxin that takes out your Iga immune system! I took all kinds of supplements, nutrients, and liver cleanses but as it turned out, I still got pneumonia. I spent a lot of time trying to unplug my liver of gallstones, some the size of 1 ½"/3 cm, but once I did that brought my health up another level. It was a chore. The patients who have severe diseases get sluggish thick bile and it turns into stones and plugs the function of your liver. This created a malfunctioning condition that backed up toxins into my body that caused me headaches and brain fog. I tried the epsom salt flush that uses oil and grapefruit juice as an emulsifier protocol to blast out stones and parasites 4x to unplug. Once the stones cleared, my energy, brain function and sense of well-being went up another level. The osteoporosis cleared itself to a point where my bone density was 20 years younger than my peers even before I unplugged my liver and started juicing. I noticed that people who juiced vegetables and fruit that were grown from soil destroyed by pesticides did not receive any health benefits, just empty colorful calories.

As a patient, I amazed the doctors who performed surgery on me, because my recovery on meal replacement was twice as fast as all the other patients. The usual follow up visits were cancelled because my recovery was so fast it didn't require them. I did almost everything outlined in this book and tried in good conscience to share the solutions with others. I never made any performance claims or charged a dollar to help anyone. With what I know now, my diseases and surgeries were irrelevant other than hard lessons learned. In every case those people with health problems who tried what I tried thrived, and those in health circumstances who didn't and followed their doctor's advice, ended up in an ambulance or fired from their jobs because of poor health unable to do their jobs.

Conclusion of examples

You cannot treat diabetes because it means you still have diabetes, you must get rid of diabetes by embracing health. You will still have susceptibility to diabetes but will be safe as long as your health is elevated. This is what they call remission, but remission really refers to a rock(s) in the bottom of your aquarium where the level of water represents your health. My point is: "instead of looking at diabetes, disease or weight gone, it is your level of health that is up". The only way to get well is to focus on the cause of what is making you unwell, and only use symptoms for diagnosis. Symptoms are just a report card of poor health.

With health problems of any kind you first want to look for symptoms of autoimmune and come down the pyramid looking at each element and how improvements can be made. There are consistent patterns for all and only a little tweaking to do for the individual with less than a dozen products for almost all disease and if you are on a budget 6 should do it. Mental illness, autoimmune, obesity and cancer require perhaps 12. For those who are healthy 1 or 2 products yield profound results.

Statistics vs Common Sense

My writer friend told me to make sure you put in a lot of statistics, readers love statistics. I was never interested in statistics for my recovery. Statistics do matter to mention because statistics are the real handicap or reason people are sick and going to stay sick. Over 90% of people with cancer go through with the recommended chemotherapy which is an oxymoron in itself because this method has less than a 10% chance of survival. Chemotherapy, radiation, surgery for cancer has been statistically proven not to work. Despite this abysmal statistical failure patients still follow the herd mentality of the sheep. You are more likely to do the wrong thing in your health care choices if you do what everyone else is doing. A lot of statistics are made up by corporate interest rather than the interest of the community anyway. Statistics that mattered to me was supplied by the autoimmune doctor, and oxygen therapy of 100% and close to it. Organic sounded right to me, not the propaganda on the TV news.

In my research I found consistent clues of information and websites to avoid. They were the websites of "official information" and of the status quo. The sites that criticize other information with facts that don't make sense and finger pointing are the sites to avoid. Their sites promoted remedies that don't work and how to cope with pain and failure to resolve health issues. With my recovery, it was risk analysis. Could it harm me if I do this or take that? Let's start with medicine vs taking a meal replacement. What are the risks with surgery to take out a gallbladder vs cleaning or flushing it? What is the risk of removing or bypassing your stomach vs cleansing your organs, and changing your diet to high density organic meal replacement and juicing vegetables? When the rheumatologist said autoimmune disease is your body's immune system attacking itself, it's confused. I said "there must be something in my body it doesn't like". This truth was realized later. I found the sites that followed a path of success without the perpetual use of drugs. Belief is the hardest part to recovery for over 99% of people I met. With persistence some come around. Money was a problem for most who wanted to try my ideas.

7 Simple Steps to health

For all these examples and for just about every disease and condition of obesity, go back to what your body needs and doesn't need with the 5 elements. Oxygen is a useful tool to pull someone from bad health. Just don't wait until you get cancer and keep this Health Handbook handy.

- You must be free from mold, and autoimmune is the most difficult condition to achieve, without help,
- Hormones infused into your blood if you are over 40, by a bioidentical hormone specialist MD is best,
- Nutrition high density meal replacement, organic fruit/vegetables, and juicing is awesome,

- Cleanse your liver and kidneys until there is no benefit, maintain a few times a year after,
- For supplements, take iodine, vitamin D 5-10,000 iu, 1 capsule of tumeric high quality, and EFA's daily, are the top inflammation reducers. Chlorella with electrolytes, aloe vera gel, apple cider vinegar together in a glass of water is awesome but not necessary every day,
- Avoid vaccination, GMO, and radiation
- Find something or someone to be passionate about. Try focusing on positive things in your life, downplay the negative as temporary. Or try reaching back to your past high lights of your life and project into the future to brighten up your future in the now.

SEQUENCE OF OBESITY & DISEASE

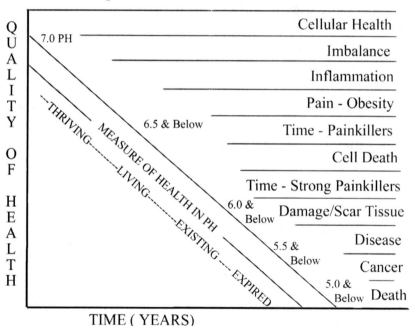

The Sequence to disease
(Down the Ladder vs Up the Ladder of Life)

CONCEPTUAL MODEL

For the future it would be helpful to adopt pH tests for everyone to help determine health of individuals. We also need to adopt the science of Fractality that could mathematically express quantitatively, Life Force energy of each food product and of each individual person. The technology is available now. Each food could have a Life Force index indicated on the label. We currently have food that has negative Life Force energy and by consuming it, will reduce your Life Force energy. There are food products that will enhance your Life Force energy when consumed.

1. CELLULAR HEALTH: The model to disease starts out as cellular health at a point of thriving. The quality of health is high and potential is realized. This is the point of super immunity and the ability to deal with stress is easy. The ease of dealing with high stress is one symptom of perfect health and "thriving".
PH is generally at 7.0-7.2 and Life force energy might be at 80% range.

2. IMBALANCE(s): This is the fulcrum point at which health changes in the sequence. It is the 2nd significant point where there is a change in the body's chemistry, a point where inflammation begins. Immunity starts to slide and problems begin to make their way into your life.
PH typically starts to slide to 6.5pH and Life force energy might be reduced to 70% range.

3. PAIN and WEIGHT GAIN: Is the 3rd significant point where physical manifestations of an imbalance in one or more of the elements of the Matrix results. It is your body's method of telling you something is wrong. Ignoring either of these symptoms has consequences. The doctors prescribe pain killers for pain and diet and exercise for obesity. The advice ignores the causes of both by not realizing the imbalances that caused either problem in the first place. Exercise puts stress on joints, adrenals and heart muscles. Diet that focuses on lowering calories increases obesity because it only increases the nutrient deficiency that leads to obesity in the first place.

A major source of pain is usually caused by nutrient deficiency and pain interferes with energy. There are layers of ailments that begin to emerge when the level of health begins to fall. Most of North Americans live at and below this level. At this level you are just "living" and not thriving and missing out on potential.

PH might be at 6.2 and a Life force at 60% range.

4. TIME: Passes, tick tock, perhaps pain killers, or the advance of diabetes, high cholesterol, or hypertension coming on? Medical drugs ignore problems and cause chemical imbalances by taking the body out of natural rhythms and puts stress on other systems leaving the stress of inflammation in the body along with cellular degeneration by not correcting the cause of the imbalance. Excess weight gain continues, quality of life declines and so does energy. Liver efficiency typically decreases.

PH might be at 6.0 and Life force at 50% range.

5. CELLULAR DEATH: With imbalances ignored, and your pain signals silenced with pain killers over time leads to cellular death, that leads to proteins in the blood settling as plaque in the brain leading to mental issues arising like dementia and permanent scar tissue beginning to set in the body and acutely in the inflamed areas. The unhealthy condition of disease and/or obesity continues its path of stress on the body leading to apathy. Oh well. Quality of life is low and health continues to decline. Your liver deteriorates from filtering toxic medicines and problems of biliary sludge forming gallstones begin to emerge as the level of water in the aquarium of life representing health continues to fall. Patients are in and out of doctor's offices and or hospitals.

PH might be about 5.8 and Life force energy at 40% range.

6. DISEASE and OBESITY: Every patient with disease has gallstones blocking proper liver function. Over time, with causes of inflammation ignored, there is a cascade of deterioration that leads to disease and perhaps organs removed. Gallbladder removal is one of the first organs to be removed and once removed is permanent and the downward spiral of apathy, low energy, and running below potential can be profound. One of the next likely organs to deteriorate is the pancreas.

PH might be down to 5.6 and Life force energy is at 30% range of just "existing".

7. CANCER is eventual unless something changes. Life is shortened, and quality of life is pathetic if left over time. Medical help is more like "life support".

PH is down below 5.4 and Life force at 1-20% range.

Ideal Health is thought to be at 6.8-7.2 pH.
Disease is thought to begin below 6.2.
Cancer is thought to begin below 5.6.
Death is thought to occur below 5.0pH.

I've known people who had blood pH of 5.0 over an extended period of time with severe disease who didn't develop cancer. It is interesting to note that the test for pH in North America of a patient is in the safe range between 4.5 and 8.0, set by the sick care system perhaps to confuse doctors and patients.

5 States the body can be in related to Life Force energy:

1. Expired in the basement of the hospital.
2. Hospitalized or institutionalized unable to cope on their own.
3. Existing, too many are hurting. Once you get sucked into the downward spiral and live in this state it is hard to get out. Finances have been drained, doctors have given up on you and some may suggest that the poor health you are experiencing is in your head. If a patient feels great they will let you know. If they were to feel ok you wouldn't find them wasting their time in a doctor's office. Unresolved problems are often referred to a mental institution which is the scrap heap of the medical system, most living in apathy with no escape.
4. LIVING, I would estimate that most of the population is just living. They need a coffee or pill to get up, a pill to get it up, they need a pill to go to sleep, they need a pill to be happy, a pill

for pain, a pill for a sniffling cold from a poor immune system. Inability to deal with stress is apparent and apathy is common.

5. THRIVING, I would estimate that a small portion of the population is realizing their potential. The euphoria of health will find a person with unstoppable energy, passion for life and fulfillment without pretending.

Thought

Sick people make sick decisions. Desperate people do desperate things. Living in these conditions man becomes more like an animal. It is a sick society that allows 50 million Americans to live without health insurance and that is old data. I believe the number is higher. 70% of people with insurance coverage go bankrupt from a health care bill. Health care in North America is like watching a train wreck in slow motion.

- I find it strange that we are not allowed to use the word "cure" when we talk about health. The true definition of "cure" is done by embracing health.
- I find it strange that the system makes it cheaper to take free meds and surgery with paid time off work, than it does to support getting healthy.
- I find it strange that one out of five kids in America are on food stamps in 2014.
- I find it strange that the doctors and scientists, the smartest people walking the earth for centuries with research money in abundance haven't found a cure for anything over the centuries? I don't consider antibiotics a cure when it shifts the problem to irritable bowel syndrome and a toxic gut where most of your immune system and central nervous system exists that lead to more disease. The statistical probability must be one in the trillions, quadrillions or more?
- I find it strange when I asked an employee who worked at a mental health clinic for 20 years, how many mental patients recovered and got off meds during your career, and she thought about it and said, "NONE".

If you get one piece of information out of these chapters that helps save someone's life out of a hundred pieces you throw away, the message will have served its purpose. The 100 pieces are in here for a reason and are responsible for holding up the floor of your health. 70% of the population is on at least one prescription medication. 70% of the North American population lives paycheck to paycheck. Consider helping others less fortunate.

There is a lot of information that flies in the face of current beliefs in these chapters because of something I call, "the normalization of nonsense".

Our system condones structure and consent of herd mentality which discourages right brain thinking and is hurting people massively. Our decisions are made by leaders who have created a system that serves their interests and not the community driven by profit. They have you believe that you are evaluated by: "the more you do, the more you are worth." The system celebrates: the more you own, what you make, and how many letters are after your name. But Law of Attraction teaches us the better you feel the more you allow. The less you know the more you understand. Tell someone how beautiful they are every day. Watch what begins to happen in your life at the realization of how to achieve health at a rate that will astonish those who surround you. Begin to Love and let go of hatred.

Summary:

The guide to lose weight in chapter 2 next, is the general guide of dos and don'ts of how to get rid of inflammation that leads to unhealthy weight. Once on the highway of health, cholesterol, diabetes, cancer, and just about every disease, and excess weight have nothing to cling to. PH and energy has nowhere to go but up. The suggestions are not weight loss suggestions, but how to embrace health. With ultimate health you will not have an unhealthy pound of weight on your body. Weight is a reflection of health and is an arbitrary number only your body will know that ultimate number.

To understand how health works, you have to focus on your health rising because you can't "beat disease". Health is like a ladder of life. Every reader can, without exception, escalate their health to a level of thriving. With the knowledge, I have no doubt that the person who needs a walker one month could be hiking up a mountain the next. The trick is acting quickly before scar tissue gets too bad and begins to deteriorate cellular integrity throughout the body.

So when the level of one's health falls, the rocks of disease and unfortunate life experiences expose themselves. By raising overall health using the 5 elements of the Matrix those exposed rocks can submerge safely below an elevated level of overall health. The exception is that health problems you are born with you will die with. Most doctors will not relate with these methods to embracing health as a solution, because they haven't been trained using these principles. They focus on the rocks of disease on the bottom of your aquarium of health, some because of belief, and some perhaps to protect their monopoly.

This book is about reaching your potential of health to the point of thriving only your body knows where to go and it can be achieved by following the information in the book. You may not initially agree at first with this information, but deep down it will plant a seed that will make sense later in an "ah-ha" moment. Knowledge is power and ignorance is bliss. Ultimate efforts yields ultimate results. You should get rid of your aching back, chronic headache, low energy, foggy memory, irritability, and perhaps increase eyesight clarity, dexterity, libido, and assume a happier disposition in life perhaps with a promotion? The suggestions that follow will increase that probability and your self-help books will begin to make more sense, if when you read them you are absent of brain fog and headaches with energy to get off the sofa and act on some good ideas!

There are two ways to be fooled. One is to believe what isn't true, and the other is to refuse to believe what is true.

To the readers and all,

I am not authorized to advise or help anyone on how to treat disease or give recommendations about health. Ideas in this book are just points to consider on your path to wellness and enlightenment. This is my story and everyone's recovery can be different in their responses to the protocols I used for myself.

The subject matter is for discussion purposes only for helping humanity realize that health care in the developed world does not exist and a new future going forward still needs to embrace the idea of treating the cause of disease and not the symptoms. When the realization that nutrition gives life and that toxins kill life, a concept society and the medical community hasn't quite yet realized, suffering of humanity can begin to subside. Many successes discussed have not been FDA assessed or peer reviewed. My belief is that this is our future of health, ideas of which are much different than the current standard. The law states that only your doctor can treat any medical condition or disease. My opinion from experience states that if your problem has anything to do with inflammation, weight loss issues or of disease that you should run. Until you experience, you won't understand why. Choosing wisely is a personal choice you must make for yourself!

How do you put a penguin into a refrigerator?
Continued chapter 2.

Chapter 2

Weight Loss

Without going hungry or the need for exercise.

Weight loss is backwards.
You can't keep fighting fires.

Weight loss is about your body needing more! Your goal should be to eat more nutrients and getting them in higher concentrations with less toxins and less waste. It's not about counting calories because your cells of your body live off nutrients. Obesity is a symptom of inflammation from an imbalance in 1 or more of the 5 elements. Someone who is obese, is probably starving to death. The body's reaction to malnutrition is to eat more. The brain scans the blood for 2 amino acids "tryptophan and glutamine". When these 2 derivatives of protein are low it triggers hunger in the brain. When EFA's (essential fatty acids) are low that triggers your craving for fats. That is why a fast food meal of 2 hamburgers, french fries and a large soda fit the bill. Sugar, fat, salt, and processed filler satisfy temporarily, but if the nutrient requirements don't fill the need from your meal, hunger comes back stronger and along with it lies the problem or "symptom" of obesity.

The problem of obesity is that it cannot be solved in a grocery store. Every product including food that is not organic sold in their isles is inflammatory, full of toxins absent of nutrients. The nutrients in every food have been removed as best as current science, and politics will permit. Obesity or excess weight is the manifestation of inflammation, period.

You will never be successful at achieving weight loss if you don't change your mind about what weight loss is. I want to repeat the message 10 different ways to de-program you. Weight loss will not give you ultimate health and getting there by starvation and exercise puts your body in stress, and lowers your energy or "Qi" of your core which hurts you.

Weight loss is about going through a checklist of what your body needs and what it doesn't need. Following the checklist helps prevent and eliminate disease and inflammation as well as unhealthy weight (muscle is healthy weight). The whole book is a checklist to achieve efficiency. For people who achieved healthy weight their ability to get off a sofa and deal with stress and symptoms of dementia declined. Again they didn't lose weight, they achieved health by eliminating inflammation. If you simply try to lose weight, and you don't lose the inflammation that caused the weight gain, sets you up for a rebound up on the bathroom scale. For some people ultimate health requires putting on weight but for most people ultimate weight is at a point somewhere lower on their bathroom scales. You have to know that muscle is heavier than fat, so vitality and shape are a better measure. Picture stomachs gone, leg and arm mass firmer and stronger, chest bigger, shoulders back. With a stronger core, liver and kidneys clean, and cells nourished, your back pain might subside, IQ and energy goes up, medicine disappears, and all your problems too. You'll have too many things going right to worry about what is wrong.

The list of "dos and don'ts" are below that will change your life.

One American Goes Bankrupt Every Second Unable to Pay Their Health Care Bill

Preamble

If you are happy with your weight loss efforts keep doing what you are doing. I was surprised to discover that excess weight is not about calories and its best to do light exercise like walking, until you get your weight down under control. Vigorous exercise is unhealthy, stressful on the heart and the adrenals when you are at an obese weight. Yo-yo dieting and exercise has not been working for as long as I can remember. I counted several different ways to lose weight and several different ways to avoid weight gain and going hungry isn't one of them. The major cause of weight gain is eating food that is rich in toxins and light on nutrients. A major way then to lose weight is to eat food that is light in toxins and rich in nutrients. Everything about achieving weight loss results in reducing inflammation. It is interesting to note that anti-inflammatory medication in the short term is contributing to obesity in the long term.

To simplify how easy it is to lose weight you should look at your body like you would your car. The regular maintenance you do on your car is to change the oil and change the filters and be sure to put clean gasoline in the tank and love is the air in your tires. How does this compare to what you are doing for your body? Your gasoline is your food for your body. Make sure your food is clear of toxins and as natural to the earth, and alive as possible and high octane organic is best to blow out the carbon. High density nutrients cool the flames of inflammation of your engine. Rust on your car is the autoimmune from having neurotoxins in your blood (chap 3). Eliminating excess weight is the same protocol to eliminating disease and thriving. The best time to quit smoking or any unhealthy addiction is when ultimate health is at an euphoric level, statistics show.

Organic is just regular food and products from 60 years ago absent of toxins with nutrients intact. Anything less will significantly compromise success of desired goals. There is nothing special about organic but compared to regular food in grocery store you are going to have problems with weight while you shop there. Note: there are many farmers growing organic fruits and vegetables without pesticides in the "ground", but it is too expensive for them to get "organic certification." That needs to change now. The major problem with non-organic is the use of pesticides in the "ground". Dead soil from pesticide use in the earth, grows dead produce, because the earth is unable to transfer nutrients to fruits and vegetables. Without the organisms alive in the earth, the nutrients are not bioavailable to the plants. That is why non-organic strawberries have no flavor or nutrients to chew on. There is about 800% more nutrients in organic produce than non-organic produce. It means that produce offered today in regular grocery stores has on average 15% of the nutrients of 60 years ago, when compared to the cross section of minerals and vitamins of produce grown with pesticides in the ground today. This is a major source of obesity. Perhaps 3 billion pounds of excess weight in North America.

For anyone who wants to improve their health and appearance, it would be great if you understood how weight loss works so that you could maximize your results. That way success is accelerated and lasting at minimal cost and time. By dieting or limiting your caloric intake the body begins to cannibalize itself by starvation and weight loss results are temporary and it's unhealthy. Weight loss for some can be achieved by simply cutting out fat food like french fries, potato chips, beer and sweets like ice cream that are low on nutrients and high in toxins and bad fats. This works by reducing the toxic burden on the health of the liver and speeding up digestion. An inefficient functioning liver is another major source of obesity.

Weight gain is one way the body expresses a health problem, the other is by pain. In the pursuit of Health, you never really have a problem, you only have an issue. Issues can be resolved. Problems only exist when you experience trauma.

The 5 elements of health that affect obesity:

All 5 elements are related to either what your body needs (nutrition) or, what your body doesn't need (toxins), similar protocol to the elimination of any disease or medication.

- Most important is ridding yourself of neurotoxins from exposure to mold. It Wreaks havoc with all systems in the body and must be removed and avoided. It is what your body doesn't need and leads to unexplainable weight gain related to the hormones leptin and cortisol, poor sleep, and low energy.
- 2nd most important is hormones. Balanced is what your body needs, like a nutrient. They are essential for cellular rejuvenation. Without them present and balanced in your blood your cells start to die, the reason for age acceleration. Proteins+amino acids+cholesterol+hormones are essential to the building blocks of cellular life.
- 3rd most important is nutrition because your cells live off nutrition. The cells are energized and repaired only through density and diversity of nutrition. The body needs 114 of these elements to thrive, 77 minerals, 18 amino acids, 3 EFA's, 16 vitamins and can

be found in 1 meal replacement. These are each like joists that hold up your floor of health. As each one goes missing, your floor starts to weaken. One is supported by the other as a symphony. You cannot get all of them through your 4 food groups. Meal replacement and trace minerals are the key along with juicing organic fruits and vegetables. Regular milk is dead of nutrients and non-organic is high on cancer causing xenoestrogens. The vitamins added are of little use to your body.

- 4th cleansing and flushing your liver and organs (of what your body doesn't need) that interfere with cellular function and nutrient absorption.
- 5th is frequency. Remove yourself from chronic toxic environments (don't need). The mind is just a processor that needs to get out of the way. Stress are just lessons and chronic stress is caused by doing the same thing over and over and expecting different results. Accept or discard each source of stress you can and find passion in the present of now or desire for the future.

There are multiple layers or sources to obesity, both primary layers as well as minor sources or "layers". To achieve ultimate weight it is best to address all sources, all the layers. The primary cause of obesity is nutrient deficiencies. People who are obese are starving to death compounded by a deactivated metabolism, along with a sick liver, hormones probably out of balance and a possibility of living in a moldy environment under stress knowing something is wrong.

In the latest example of medical insanity, we're now learning that an obese two-year-old child has been subjected to bariatric surgery.

Cutting out part of your stomach, or surgery to bypass is an unfortunate solution and not necessary. If you are going to lose weight you need to do it with some intensity and be commited to flush out toxins and infuse your cells with nutrients. The drip of a healthy meal here and there will not do it, but an effort more like the flush of a fire hose is more like it. With an abundance of healthy high density nutrients and juicing starves unhealthy weight. Nutrients take about 10-14 days to permeate throughout your cells, where you begin to notice significant change of your skin health. The liver flush by Isagenix.com, gives you a deep cellular cleanse like no other I have come across and will give you fast results if your liver is unplugged. I found the only significant way to clean your liver was to starve it of nutrients for 2 days. The Isagenix liver cleanse works with natural ingredients like an emulsifier on toxic chemicals and fats in the liver for elimination, promoting increased efficiency right down the digestive tract. Follow by drinking 12 oz. glasses of organic juiced vegetables daily. Organic vegetables are a major deficiency of North Americans and are considered carbohydrates. You will notice your energy and eyesight improve within 30 minutes of consumption.

The goal is not to lose weight but to embrace health and healthy weight will follow automatically. Awesome weight is a function of awesome health absent of inflammation.

LADDER OF LIFE CHART
Life Force energy of you as a reflection of potential. I went from close to 0% hospitalized in a wheelchair for a year to 70% rollerblading, going to the gym and bench pressing 150% of my weight for 10 repetitions.

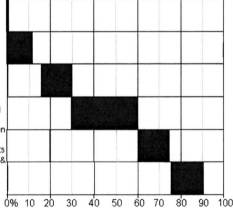

Death

Hospitalized, cancer, acute disorders, multiple drugs & symptoms, unable to work For 7% of population.

Existing with obesity, diabetes, tired before, during, after work. Work performance marginal. Punching a clock at work & in life. For 40% pop.

Living on coffee, pills for sleep, headaches, tired after work. Average existence and ability to deal with stress. Uninspired. For about 30% population

Living & eating organic, excercising/gym workouts Above average performance dealing with stress & work.

Thriving from meal replacements, juicing, excercising. Thrives at work, home & with stress

0% 10 20 30 40 50 60 70 80 90 100

With excess weight eliminated you can then push your body with a cardio routine that will respond with results that will impress. Inflammation drains your energy because your body's resources focus on resolving inflammation. As a consequence your body puts less energy into other bodily functions that aren't important. Autoimmune patients should avoid exercise because it accelerates damage to your body because of neurotoxins circulating in the blood that exacerbates inflamed tissue instead of repairing similar to the way water reacts to rust. That is why your hands, knees and to a lesser extent hips get inflamed and damaged. Celiac, crohn's, colitis, and IBS (irritable bowel syndrome) are on the increase because of trying to digest toxic GMO and new chemicals in food. With GMO's present, inflammation is focused to your digestive tract for a neurotoxin assault while you digest food that is inflammatory. For others, the muscles used the most during gardening and walking when neurotoxins are present intensifies inflammation to those areas.

We will never get out of the rut of ill health and ill weight if you remain stuck in beliefs from the last centuries.

Food allergies, food sensitivities, edema and for some asthma, are symptoms of toxic overload from a sick liver full of gallstones, you need to flush repeatedly and clean repeatedly (see Chapter 6 cleansing). If you weren't born with it, you don't need to live with it or die with it. The water retention you experience in your body and ankles are symptoms of toxic overload in your cells and your body's response is to dilute the toxicity with swelling. Do not take water pills to reduce the water retention it only increases toxin concentrations.

Water retention is caused by an imbalance in the equation of toxin in and toxins eliminated and the result is inflammation.

It is a natural warning that the medical community ignores. Your body is perfect and our world is not. A major health objective is to reduce toxins in your body. Further down are about 40 ways to do that.

Healthy weight loss was about 3/4th of a pound a day over 60 days without going hungry or exercising for as many days as it took to achieve healthy weight. For the impatient, the fastest way to lose weight is by cleaning your liver first. I had people lose 12 unhealthy lbs. after completion of a single two day Isacleanse a week later. Weight loss comes a week later, as a result of an improved functioning liver and has nothing to do with calorie equations. It's not about diet and exercise. When you clean your liver there are several other benefits of health that are experienced including improved immunity. Once you are free of neurotoxin concerns and your choice of nutrients are top notch, and your filters are clean, you need to focus on your gut flora with probiotics to get those nutrients absorbed with maximum efficiency. Gut flora is sacred and your power comes from there. It is destroyed by fast food and toxins in food your body doesn't recognize along with GMO's.

Over time the body is worn down slowly into the ground on a daily basis in the form of malnutrition, toxins from a poor diet, poor gut flora (candida) and this contributes to an inability to deal with stress. The result of how you deal with stress can be a compromised immune system, lowering of the IQ and shrinking of overall ability to deal with stress and lack of energy. Inflammation begets inflammation, being fat begets being more fat, and being stressed begets more stress. All are a multi-symptom cocktail of imperfection that has become more common recently in society today with 75,000 chemical toxins that have been introduced into the food chain, air and water and the extraction of nutrients from just about everything you eat.

Reminding you that, finding food in a grocery store that isn't fattening, that contributes to a diseased body is almost impossible. If you want to be healthy don't buy anything from a store unless it is organic or at the very least has been grown without the use of pesticides in the soil. You should familiarize yourself with the serial number stuck on organic fruit and vegetables beginning with a 9, or buy from a farmer who will be honest about not growing with pesticides in the ground. Support your farmers and their fight against Monsanto. Family farmers are the people suffering the most with their battles against Monsanto's ruthless assault on healthy food and those who grow it while you are at work. Give to Farm Aid.

The body is a perfect machine. It came from a single cell and knew what to do and how to grow itself into a physical body with blood, tissue, bone, eyes, heart, and a brain, to thrive in the absence of poison and in the presence of nutrition during gestation. The body can be brought back to that state of perfection aside from scar tissue at any time during one's life.

Life expectancy for a human is 120 years old. That means playing tennis when you are 100. Dr. Gerson lived to age 117 using his method of juicing nutrients out of fruits and vegetables, throwing out the worthless pulp and using a coffee detox.

Methods to lose Weight dos and don'ts
All are anti-inflammatory, anti-disease, anti-dementia, pro health and immunity, pH alkaline

Nutrients
It's not about calories because your body doesn't live off calories, it craves and lives off nutrients. To address the issue properly you must look at the quality or nutrient density and Life Force energy. I found it with meal replacement of 114 essential nutrients. I didn't need to learn about nutrition because you won't get healthy from eating from the 4 food groups. That means about the equivalent of 10 meals of nutrients in one glass of water with less than 500 calories. When you meet nutrient demands you no longer have hunger. Hunger comes from nutrient deficiency. To meet nutrient demands with high density, the other most effective methods is juicing vegetables and fruits. Both absorb into the blood stream as fast as alcohol without being compromised by the digestive tract. Wow. Below are other ideas:

FRUIT: I made smoothies, I ate organic fruit, and had a container of fruit meal replacement on my counter to add to the fruits I blended. The seeds from fruit are a raw form of laetrile (a B17 vitamin) which kills cancer cells on contact. Food from the earth is perfect.

For PROTEIN: I had meal replacement of 2 types in canisters on the kitchen counter or for trips on the seat of my car. I would have 2 scoops in one glass daily that would give me 18 amino acids, fibre, minerals and vitamins, the equivalent to 10 meals of nutrients in one glass from Isashake from Isagenix.com. Isashake got me out my wheelchair in 2 weeks after being atrophied for close to 2 years, without physio or exercise. This mixture shocked my surgeons regarding my speedy recovery. I also use a blend that is not commercially available that is hand-made and about 50%

more effective with non-processed ingredients, that is spectacular. That product unfortunately is not commercially available.

For GREENS: I had containers of Progressive of Canada, and Vega meal replacement,

JUICING: I juiced organic beets, apples, cucumbers, carrots, celery, kale and drank 12-16 oz per day. The results of drinking this juice was as amazing as doing meal replacements are.

GREEN SUPPLEMENTS: I had a pail of chlorella, spirulina, alfalfa I would add to either the Greens meal replacement or make into a tincture with aloe vera gel, cinnamon, ginger, electrolytes for hydration, and apple cider vinegar in a glass of water. Chlorella and spirulina are also detoxifying of heavy metals. They are great for mental illness because both cross the blood brain barrier for detoxification of the brain as well as throughout the body. Profound relief of those who suffered from a regular food diet by drinking my aloe vera tincture was about 30 minutes. This tincture is great for college students following a drinking party.

SNACKS: For snacks air popping organic corn kernels and melting coconut oil with Himalayan sea salt is awesome and healthy. Baking kale chips in the oven with Himalayan sea salt is a great replacement for potato chips. Applying by hand coconut oil or virgin oil to each leaf prior to baking helps with flavor. Organic cheese/humus and crackers, or organic corn chips with flax seed, organic coconut ice cream bars are ideas.

For SUPPLEMENTS:

- take 8-10,000 iu of vitamin D on days you aren't in the sun, more on D in chapter 8,
- Iodine daily, women should take a double dose it is important you do,
- EFA's daily, cuts down the cravings for bad fats (omega 3, 6, 9's),
- Tumeric 1 tablet daily of high quality to lower inflammation in 30 minutes,
- Probiotics daily maintenance for superior nutrient absorption,

For THOSE WITH DISEASE add:

- Larch tree extract for cancer and autoimmune conditions, lowers TNF-b1
- Glutathione is powerful antioxidant for liver diseases and cancer. It is dispensed in natural path's offices by intravenous for inflammation relief. I will try to get a non-commercial brand together that I use which is economical at 1/50th the cost of getting it by IV. Until then there is a product by Max International that incorporates N-acetyl cysteine formula that enables your body to make glutathione at the cellular level that is sold in a canister.

FOOD from the KITCHEN: I would have 1 meal a day of something organic. I cooked with coconut oil in the fry pan. It is healthy for the brain and doesn't break down with heat into toxic substances. Organic soups are sold at the health food store, the only place you should buy your food for the kitchen.

Tea: I would occasionally make parsley water tea that would give relief to kidney pain within 12 hours of drinking the first mug. You can mix this as cool water in with your meal replacement for extra awesome health benefits. The tea has a refrigerator life of about a week max.

SALAD/VEGETABLES: I tried to have daily.

The ideal portion of your diet should be about 40% vegetables and consider juicing. Cooking kills nutrients so be gentle, perhaps steam them. By juicing you get a large amount of nutrients absorbed into the blood as fast as alcohol in only 15 minutes without the nutrient destruction of going through your digestive tract. Juicing your vegetables has an added effect of detoxifying your liver and the cells in your body.

About 30-40% of your diet should be protein I got from meal replacement and 20-30% fiber. The good meal replacements will have 24 grams of protein, 8 grams of dietary fiber, and have dozens of vitamins, minerals and contain digestive enzymes with probiotics to aid and speed up digestion also helping nutrient absorption. They will also have 18 amino acids that are necessary for cellular reproduction. It is proteins and cholesterol, amino acids, with hormones balanced, that makes for a cocktail of perfection for cellular rejuvenation. The combination improves the life force energy of everyone including vegetarians or vegans within 10-14 days. Meal replacements are a relief to a worn out body because they are absent of toxins, GMO, artificial color or artificial flavors. An active carpenter can take 2 scoops in the morning of a meal replacement and move around tons of lumber and pound in a box of nails and make it to lunch without feeling hungry, with unusually high energy within a few days of starting the meal replacement. Results speak louder than words. I talked an acquaintance into using a meal replacement and cleansing his liver, and he said his hair got thicker, vision improved, he lost 40 lbs, his nails got harder, skin color healthier, he could think clearer, sex drive went up and he had unbelievable energy. This is similar to the symptoms of someone on Bio available hormones. Another benefit of meal replacement is that it reduces visceral fat which is dangerous fat that settles around your organs.

High protein and amino acids are important because your brain triggers hunger by scanning the blood for the proteins, Tryptophan and Glutamine. Healthy EFA's are essential fatty acids that trigger cravings for "fat" foods. Your body is smarter than any doctor.

Trace minerals sold at a health food store will give you the 77 minerals your body is looking for. When these are low, the quickest way to satisfy hunger is by eating calories rich in sugar, salt, and fat. The salt and fat from potato chips and a sweet tasting soda or chocolate bar typically answer the craving temporarily but compounds the problem because hunger not satisfied with nutrients will come back stronger than ever, while a few more pounds settle around your abdomen while you are waiting.

To find out how our food is being adulterated, watch the movie "Super Size Me" or "Food Inc" on Youtube.com. The trouble with fast food is that it is a temporary fix for your craving and leaves your body starving for nutrients. Fast food is dispensed out of a window and is absent of nutrients, rich in unhealthy fat, flavored by salt and sugar which further compounds the problem of obesity. Because your body doesn't recognize what it has consumed, it sits in your gut, slows your digestion and plugs up your liver of toxins and fats, which is another major cause of obesity in itself. I just counted 3 sources of obesity and disease by eating fast food: High toxins, low nutrients, and slowed digestion. Slowed digestion is caused by a lack of bioavailability of the fast food, which means your body doesn't recognize what it is trying to digest.

- If your BELLY PROTRUDES out from your belt, it is a symptom of a sick, toxic, fat inefficient liver. Expect it to be plugged with gallstones, which is the primary cause of hypertension, asthma, allergies, food allergies, chemical sensitivity and is the secondary cause of bad cholesterol in your blood tests. If you are over 40, another layer of fat develops because of low hormones.
- If your BELLY STICKS OUT AND DROPS BELOW YOUR BELT and your arms are flabby you will also have an improper ratio of good to bad bacteria, in your gut, which leads to slow digestion and poor nutrient absorption. The answer is probiotics and digestive enzymes with high density food.
- If you are GENERALLY OVER WEIGHT, and diet and exercise aren't working, this is usually an under active thyroid caused by low iodine along with the 2 conditions mentioned above. Iodine is bleached out of body by drinking and bathing in municipal tap water that has chlorine or fluoride added. Both are about as toxic as arsenic, both are cumulative and both have no benefit to human life in any way and should be left as industrial waste in China where it came from. Hypothyroidism and MRSA, now are at epidemic rates, are primarily caused by low iodine. The thyroid when it is properly functioning filters bacteria in your blood like a UV filter that cleans your water of bacteria.

A lot of books are being sold hyping phyto-nutrients, they will contribute to Super Immunity, but will not give you Super Immunity alone, perhaps only a 30% by contribution and perhaps only10% when hormones and neurotoxins are considered in overall health, and 0% contribution to super immunity, if the phyto-nutrients are non-organic. Phyto-nutrients aren't nearly as good unless they are organic. The scientific reports that are not bought and paid for show that organic fruits and vegetables have 800% more nutrients in them, than non-organic. Just compare an organic strawberry to a non-organic strawberry grown with pesticides if you don't believe me.

There is food, then there is food byproduct and then worse, there is food replacement. GMO food cannot be considered food because it has a negative Life Force energy that actually hurts you by consuming it. An example of a food byproduct is pasteurized milk that is heated up to the point where the nutrients are cooked out of it and now, there is Ultra-pasteurized milk which makes it "ultra" non-nutritional and the vitamins they add have no significant nutritional value to you similar to what they do with iodine and salt. Raw milk untreated, is extremely rich in nutrients and in my opinion the only healthy version of cow milk there is. It is illegal to sell raw milk in North America and there are more and more farmers who are currently facing criminal charges for drinking and selling their own raw milk. Raw organic milk has a shelve life of 10-14 days refrigerated and should be the only milk sold in stores. There is a farmer in Oregon with a 100+ acres who was recently arrested and thrown in jail for collecting rain water. Rain is subject to a law that gives the water commission full ownership and rights that has no consideration to the property owner. Water is the new oil of the future. Unless your food is grown without pesticides in the ground, it cannot be considered food, but a food byproduct that contributes to obesity.

Chemical food dependency Vs the Euphoria of Health from Raw Wholesome Food

A drug or chemical food addiction like coffee is hard to break but perhaps can be broken by focusing on achieving the euphoria of health. If you can consume an ideal diet for a week or two and go back to your old unhealthy diet of chemical dependency, it will make you sick and give you stomach cramps and remind you why you need to switch your diet back to a healthy one. I gave a friend a half liter/quart of juiced vegetables and apples in the morning and she couldn't eat dinner at her favorite restaurant that night, it made her feel sick to eat GMO pasta. A good juicer can be bought for 200$ or 80$ used. No one can afford to be sick.

To try and motivate yourself back to health, try standing outside an organic store then stand outside a discount grocery store for 10 minutes and assess each patron's physical condition. You can also motivate yourself if you put a hot body of someone you would like to be or be with or look like on your fridge. Wealth, romance, abundance and self-love come from a healthy body, and a healthy mind. I can see problems eating organic food that is foreign to your taste buds at the beginning but you will notice how good you feel, with clear mind, energy, and pain starting to leave your body, before you go back to a jumbo bag of potato chips with dip. More on nutrients in Chapter 5.

The most important nutrients are the ones that you are missing.

IODINE is in every cell in your body or should be. Development of proper brain function and high IQ in children are from: iodine, the animal based omega 3 fat DHA, vitamin D, avoiding fluoride, and optimizing gut flora. Iodine moves nutrients into and cellular waste out of each living cell in your body. It is the most single important nutrient the entire adult population in the developed world is critically deficient in. The statistic is 97% because the other 3% already supplement. It is the supplement you need when you can't lose weight with diet and exercise. For that reason it is the most important weight loss/ disease-freeing supplement there is. The effects on weight and inflammation when this is low are immense. One of the primary functions of the thyroid is metabolism regulation. It does this by affecting the mitochondria inside the cells. Your metabolic rate determines whether you gain or lose weight. Your thyroid can't function properly if it doesn't have enough iodine to make the thyroid hormone. When your body's metabolism slows down you get cold feet and hands and you get muscle cramps at night and gain weight.

Typical table salt is not salt but poison that tastes like salt. To suggest that salt contains enough iodine to maintain healthy levels is criminal. So many factors are not considered. In the manufacturing process of salt, it is heated to 1100F to a point where the molecules are rearranged such that the body does not recognize table salt. It is not bioavailable to your body which means your body doesn't recognize it. What your body doesn't recognize is not life sustaining and what is not life sustaining is poison. This processed unnatural type of salt, contributes to hypertension and obesity which is a symptom of a sick liver filtering poison out of your blood beyond capacity. Salt is essential for making stomach acid to break down proteins into amino acids and without it you develop allergies to protein. Salt is essential to a healthy body and you need to go to a health food store to get real salt. Regulations allow for salt sold in grocery stores to be labeled "sea salt" with as little as 8% content. The balance of the 92% can be the type that is processed and toxic to your body.

Himalayan sea salt taken every day and a triple dose of iodine, in my opinion for months for nutrient loading of iodine and a daily dose for the rest of your lives is essential. To stop the bleaching of your iodine out of your body place a filter on your shower heads and stop drinking tap water. Better yet, stop putting fluoride or chlorine in the municipal water supply, this is not potable water worthy for livestock. Livestock that drink natural non-toxic water will drink more, yield more, be healthier and have lowered vet bills. To encourage natural iodine intake we need to stop the pesticide application on crops that kill the soil and try to grow your own fruits and vegetables in your backyard or buy organic.

The presence of iodine in your body from supplements, food supply and a clean water supply to preserve inventory of iodine, will stimulate your metabolism and solve hypothyroidism, and a couple of dozen health ailments. Farmers are the healthiest in the country who live absent of fluoride and pesticides on their farms. Iodine paired up with Iodide is the most bio-available source and when added with Selenium and B2 optimizes activation of the thyroid. This combination is about 800% more bioavailable than potassium iodine. A more effective form of potassium iodine, is potassium iodide called Lugol's developed in 1829 in France and found at most local drug stores if you ask for it. Iodine is most prominent in thyroid and breast tissue and also important in brain, stomach, ovaries, salivary glands and your eyes. Women need more because breast tissue needs so much iodine. Normal levels of iodine are essential for women to be fertile, with levels too low there is an off switch flipped for fertility. Taking iodine during pregnancy improves their baby's IQ. Women have persistent baby fat around their tummies following birth because they give up half their iodine to their baby. It deactivates their metabolism so exercise to remove baby fat around the middle will almost be impossible. Selenium is necessary for the iodothyronine deiodinase enzyme to properly function. It is critical to enhance conversion of T4 into T3 which is the active hormone of your thyroid. Riboflavin or vitamin B2 has been shown to help the body make proper amounts of active thyroid hormones. Iodine assists cell metabolism and energy.

The symptoms of low iodine from fluoride/chlorine in the water:

- Weight Gain	- Difficulty losing weight	- Low energy
- Cold (always feeling cold)	- Ice cold hands or feet	- Dry skin
- Hair loss	- Poor concentration slow thought	- Poor sleep
- Brain fog	- Memory problems	- Waking up tired
- Tingling hands and feet	- Muscle aches	Edema - Swelling ankles
- Constipation	- Slow heart rate	- thick tongue
- Low iron in blood	- Thinned eyebrows	- Muscle cramps at night
- Slow reflexes	- Skin itches in winter	- Regular headaches
- Decreased sweating	- Problems getting pregnant	- Pale puffy skin
- Decreased body hair	- Dizziness	- Hoarse voice

SUPPLEMENTS:

- Vitamin D is involved in over 2000 metabolic activities in the body and is an anti-inflammatory. Vitamin D doesn't start working until you take a minimum of 5000iu/day, but 8-10,000iu is best. Vitamin D also works to eliminate menstrual cramps in 30 minutes and is good for you. Sitting in the midday sun (best without burning) for an hour with as much exposed skin and without suntan lotion will give you 10,000iu of Vitamin D synthesis to reduce inflammation and weight throughout your body. It is the the 2nd most important supplement for losing weight, lowering inflammation and staying healthy provided you meet the minimum 5000iu daily in concentration dose for it to work.

-   Tumeric is also anti-inflammatory. It is a spice from India used in cooking. It reduces inflammation within 30 minutes. Because these 2 supplements are anti-inflammatory, they are also anti-cancer, anti-obese, anti-disease supplements. Taking these supplements will help with weight loss but do have a minor effect.

LIVER CLEANSE: Is a major way to lose weight especially around the middle. It is the 4th most important element to achieve health and weight loss when you bring your liver back to life. Medical blood tests do not reliably test for sick livers until it is too late. Just look to see if you have a belly that sticks out and you probably have an inflamed fatty liver that isn't working properly. Cleaning your liver every week until there is no benefit is what it takes. Weight loss or I like to call it, loss of inflammation occurs mostly with the belly but throughout the body as well. It can take several weekends, but cleaning your liver should reduce or eliminate high blood pressure, allergies, chemical sensitivity and asthma. It will also help to improve energy, depression, dementia, immunity, IQ, libido, luck, and vibration. This is one of the top ways to lose weight but requires the most effort and attention to detail. Before you clean your liver you should unplug it with an Epsom salt flush to clear blockages which is harder on the body and should not be done anything less than 2 weeks apart. That method goes back thousands of years. There is another method that can remove gallstones, is more expensive, but is useful for those that have had their gallbladders removed or who are weak from disease, or are elderly. The method dissolves the stones using Chanca Piedra a supplement from Peru, rather than flushing stones to get the liver working properly.

HORMONES: Hormones balanced to levels of a 30 year old by using a Bio-Identical Hormone specialist MD is an ideal way to lose unhealthy weight or to put on healthy weight and is the 2nd most important way to achieve optimum health. Hormones are important and are like the computer software of the body. 50 mg of DHEA daily, for males with the option of taking testosterone, 3 weeks on and one week off a month seems to be ideal to keep your own testosterone production going, but consult your doctor. Testosterone is not optional unless it is taken with DHEA. For females progesterone daily and estrogen is optional, perhaps 3 weeks a month might be your ideal option. Women menstruating can just take progesterone on the last 15 days of your cycle and for post-menopausal women you can take it daily. Estrogen should be a reduced dose because it is so prevalent in plastics, underarm deodorant, and in regular laundry detergent, but consult with your Bio-Identical Hormone specialist MD not your doctor. I found that your family doctor has not had enough training to express a safe opinion for such an important topic. Hormones work great when you are over 40 and most effective over the age of 50. After 35 the adult hormones begin to fall off and as a result you begin to lose about a pound a year of muscle. The aging process begins when collagen production and cellular rejuvenation in relation to cellular death begins to fall. With the presence of hormones the process of cell rejuvenation accelerates. That's why kids who have optimal hormones can play soccer, eat toxic fast food and still have energy. I talked to people who used Amberen who experienced success for menopause relief for, hot flashes, weight control, irritability, sleeplessness and other symptoms of menopause. A four week treatment with Amberen increased the level of estradiol fourfold in menopausal women. Estrogen supplementation on its own is of risk for cancer when it is not opposed to progesterone.

CARDIO should be done in the morning because it stimulates the metabolism. The calories burned during a 12 minute session of exercise continues to burn throughout the day. People who can't lose weight from exercising will have iodine levels that are too low from an under active metabolism and a malfunctioning liver. Cardio exercise has benefits of anaerobic cell elimination through the introduction of oxygen into the cells and blood, as well as toxin elimination by sweating through your pores. The jarring action and agitation of cells massages toxins out of cells for elimination. Cardio also increases oxygen exchange efficiency in the capillaries of the lungs and improves IQ levels by up to 10%, lowers the stress hormone levels of Cortisol and increases mood with secretion of endorphins from the brain, and bone density improves because pH is raised. Regular cardio jogging with intensity spurts is recommended.

Marathon running is not good for you and shortens life expectancy because of the stress on your body and exposes nutrients that are lacking that are not being replaced through diet. Consuming a high density protein shake meal replacement within 30 minutes of a workout is necessary for muscles to repair following exercising. If you are going to a gym it is best to do high repetition with low weight to tone muscles not build them. You should drink a glass of water (non-toxic) following exercise to eliminate toxins through urine following a workout.

PROBIOTICS help you maximize nutrient absorption of what you eat and are very important. They are good for displacing unhealthy anaerobic bacteria which causes yeast in your gut. A history of a poor diet is helped with a daily dose of probiotics. The consumption of probiotics will reduce abdominal bloating, help with Irritable Bowel Syndrome. A good probiotic can make a difference to your health. The probiotic I am thinking of has a 3 year shelf life with no refrigeration and seems to be 10x more effective than anything I've tried in stores. The superior probiotic that worked for me seemed to give me an iron gut. Be aware that about a 1/3rd of probiotics tested and sold in stores were found to be dead on arrival on your kitchen counter. I would recommend buying all your supplements from a health food store that specializes in quality nutrients where nutrients are maximized and toxins are minimized. The less time your body spends sorting through usable nutrients from the unusable toxins for elimination the better health you will be. Your body will reward you when you reward it, bringing you closer to ideal weight.

ENZYMES make digestion efficient when combined with probiotics. Digestive enzymes make the nutrients in your food bio-available to your cells. They break down the nutrients in your food to a state in which your body can readily absorb. When you eat regular human food at a restaurant, not to be mistaken with organic fruit and vegetables and meal replacements, you need digestive enzymes added. So the nutrients from any regular home cooked meal or meal on the road would benefit with a pill or 2 of digestive enzymes which you can buy from a health food store. This one supplement has a minimal effect on weight loss but, if you have soft fat or IBS disease, this is where it will help most. Soft fat is a symptom of slow digestion. Meal replacements only cost 1 or 2 dollars a serving and usually have the digestive enzymes and probiotics in each serving.

FLUSH/ACCELERATOR are 2 products sold by Isagenix.com intended for weight loss and helpful most for soft fat weight loss by speeding up digestion. I use the accelerator and flush product to speed up the digestion of unhealthy food when I eat something that tastes good but has no nutrient value like poutine (fries/gravy/cheese). My stomach looks at the mess of calories and says: "What tis this?" Raw food is food that is alive high in nutrient concentration and is bio-available which means your body loves it! What your body loves, your body responds well to, and will love you. "Natural or fresh" food usually means put it back on the shelf.

GRAZING and SMALL FREQUENT MEALS contribute to weight loss. Slow continuous feeding is more effective than a feast. Eating a big meal, high in protein in the morning and tapering off during the day is best. You get maximum utility throughout the day when your metabolism is highest and when your body needs nutrition the most. Metabolism is lowest at night when you are at rest. Overeating, even healthy food, will make us lethargic as the digestive system sucks energy from other organs to digest the extra food and slows down digestion which is fattening in itself.

TAOIST DIET can take you down 5 lbs. in 30 days if you try to follow it. The first practice is to always have fruit on its own. Fruit has a digestion cycle of 20 minutes so eat it first. Protein and Carbs conflict with one another but each can be eaten with vegetables and or salads. Avoid smoking, coffee, alcohol, soda within ½ hour of eating, and drink room temperature water or beverages so as not to coagulate the fats in your stomach of the food you are eating, it slows digestion and contributes to weight gain. Ice water or soda will solidify the fat in your food slowing digestion and impeding nutrient absorption.

JUICING is an awesome way to get high density live food nutrients to the cells and when combined with meal replacements for protein it is even more awesome because the juice is delivered to the cells as fast as alcohol. It is superior method to get nutrition that avoids the digestive tract and delivers nutrients unharmed in perfect preservation to your cells. Not only is it superior nutrition but also over time allows detoxification of the organs and cells. Juicing organic is mandatory for thriving. The waste pulp properly juiced from a Gerson Juicer has no nutritional value and to prove it the used pulp from your juicer from a bag of carrots will be rejected by your horses. Just convert your vegetables to juice as you need it because it spoils quickly in the fridge.

LEPTIN pay attention to Leptin. It is a protein hormone that plays a key role in regulating energy intake and expenditure including appetite and hunger. Leptin becomes out of balance in patients who are auto-immune and that triggers hunger. Leptin acts on receptors in the hypothalamus of the brain, where it inhibits appetite.

SLEEP is the best healer there is, and is key to finding a healthy weight. Releasing spasm from the body is a key to sleeping well. Massage, sex, sensible sun exposure, and jogging release spasm from the body. I found that sleep deprivation is caused by spasm in the body, and when it is released, sleep and the healing effects from it come easy. There is a whole host of causes for spasm to accumulate in the body and its consequence is sleep debt. Sleep debt means you can actually store sleep which is unhealthy and one of the symptoms very often, is weight gain, compromised immunity and inability to deal with stress. Deep sleep reduces the stress hormone cortisol, so does laughter, and exercise.

Other ways to get sleep:

- Melatonin in pill form, you dissolve under your tongue before bed. It is natural to the body safe to use long term, 3 and 5 mg.
- Blackout your windows, tin foil works well and blocks out heat
- Sleep in temperatures below 70F or 21C
- Remove clocks and phones away from your head
- TV, Ipads, and computers that emit light suppresses natural melatonin secretion in your body, and lowers male fertility
- Sleeping pills don't work well and interfere with brain function during waking hours.

- Regular sleep patterns help establish healthy weight and energy. Shift workers should get 20 minutes of sun in their faces before falling asleep after coming off shift work because the sun is a natural reset mechanism for your biological clock.
- Discover ear plugs, they work great to block out a chance siren going by at night.
- Sunshine in your face and on your skin is great!

SUNSHINE is a way to lose weight. It is the UVB rays of the midday sun that heals your body and is anti-inflammatory and allows you to get deep restful sleep. The deep penetrating rays will take spasm out of your body and at the same time remove inflammation and increase your energy. The conversion of sun rays to Vitamin D has a profound healing effect with over 2000 metabolic functions going on in the body. In Chicago/Toronto about 44'N of the equator (the sun moves1.8'/weekly), the UVB is present midday at 1 pm from April 1 to Sept 15. It is the late day and early morn UVA sun that ages the skin. Avoid wearing suntan lotion if you can as the lotion stops the conversion of the suns rays to vitamin D. Make sure the lotion is Organic from a health food store where the ingredients are not poison and are as close to natural and therefore harmless to your body, if you have to wear it. Lotion should only be used to avoid burning because suntans are healthy. The rays from the sun actually prevent almost all cancer and the non-organic lotions cause the skin cancer. Not only do the non-organic lotions contain poisons, but they block out the healing rays of the sun while those poisonous ingredients are absorbed into the blood stream, a double whammy. The absorption happens much the same way as a hormone prescription filled from a pharmacy is rubbed into your skin through the fat layer and later migrating into the blood stream.

The studies indicate that the closer to the equator people are, the less skin cancer happens. The farther north you get the higher the incidence of skin cancer. These studies indicate that cancer is not caused by the sun. Adding suntan lotion and staying out of the midday sun only increases that statistic of disease. Expose as much skin to the sun as possible for the healing healthy effects. Avoid wearing sunglasses when possible, it is better for you than wearing them. There are streams of energy that your eyes absorb when you are not wearing sunglasses by means of ambient light. Some people look into the sun at sunset and sunrise to absorb the atmosphere-filtered sun to absorb the streams of energy, but this should be practiced with caution. For shift workers the sun helps reset your biological clock, so if you are working shifts or out late partying and come out into the morning sun it is best to sit and face the sun with your eyes closed for 20 minutes. This will give you a great sleep and help take the spasm out of your body following exposure.

Sunshine also zaps the zits out of teenagers and all ages by drying out the excess oils in the skin. Next time you pull out your suntan lotion look at the ingredients. If they are 26 letters long and have a lot of X's and Y's in them with words you don't recognize and neither does anyone you know, throw it in the garbage. If you can't eat what you are putting on your skin don't put it on your skin. The chemicals cause cancer and plug up your liver with poisons which contributes to obesity by reducing the efficiency of your liver. I've read that some of the ingredients in suntan lotion intensify their toxicity with exposure to the sun when applied to the skin. If this is true this is evil science on steroids. Sunshine gives relief to autoimmune patients and makes them feel better and more energetic with less spasm. The radiant heat from the sun detoxifies the blood and brings down swelling in joints and tissue. If you don't believe me ask the people coming home from a winter in the desert or notice how good you feel after a nice summer of sun.

ELECTROLYTES in your water bottle is awesome for hydration and getting rid of leg cramps. You can actually dehydrate from drinking too much water. The hydration drinks sold in the convenience stores have too many toxins and HFCS is a primary cause of cholesterol. I read that there are only 2 nutrients in Gator Aid.

Inflammatory Sources - Disease A-Z
That Create Symptoms of Obesity, Inflammation and disease and poor immunity

    a.   PASTEURIZED FOOD is absent of nutrients. The heat process cooks the nutrient value out of the food and is referred to as a food byproduct. An example is milk and most yogurt. Most yogurt listing probiotic bacteria as an ingredient usually doesn't have live cell probiotics in them even though they advertise that on the label. Organic yogurt is most likely to have probiotics alive, with healthy nutrients inside without the sugars that makes you fat, nor the "fat-free" processing that removes nutrients. Removing nutrients also makes you fat.

b. TABLE SALT is mislabeled because it is poison that tastes like salt. Poison that doesn't kill you creates obesity by reducing the efficiency of the liver filtering the toxins. Salt also contributes to hypertension. Hypertension is a symptom of a sick liver. There is virtually no beneficial iodine in salt, so take iodine supplement from your local health food store for life literally.

c. BIO-AVAILABILITY OF NUTRIENTS is so important. Does your body recognize the substance as food? The more bio-available the nutrient the more life sustaining it is. Life sustaining food has an alkalizing effect on the pH of the blood. Eating alkaline food and water does not make you alkaline it is the Life Force energy of the food absent of chemicals that will make you alkaline. Theoretically alkaline water will make you more acidic than natural water not processed in its natural form. You can buy water attachments for industrial and home use that incorporate the spin vortex of fractality to increase Life Force energy of your water that comes out the tap. A strawberry field watered with this commercial application yielded 30% more strawberries from the same acreage as the field watered by regular distribution without filtration, one field being adjacent to the other. Several feet out from the sprayed area also benefitted by this spun water without there being ever any physical contact with the spun water. This is amazing technology of Life Force energy in practice. The home attachment is about $299.

d. MOLD has a devastating effect on the body. Autoimmune, like no other disease and is a major source of problems that also lead to weight gain because of an increase in Leptin. There are so many negative symptoms of autoimmune. This is caused by living or working in toxic moldy living conditions wreaking havoc with hormones and energy levels.

e. AVOID ASPARTAME food that is diet anything. Aspartame is the feces or excrement of E-Coli, a Cytotoxin that creates holes in the brain and later turns to embalming fluid in the body. Approved or allowed by consent by the FDA after decades of being rejected as poison by ethical science. Toxins impede proper function of the liver thus contributing to obesity more than regular soda. Similarly, diet food is more processed thus having its nutrients reduced that causes obesity.

f. FAT FREE means processed which means shallow or absent of nutrients. Fats like your Omega 3, 6, 9 are actually good for your brain and skin. Avoid anything with zero calories on the label.

g. AVOID SHOPPING in a GROCERY STORE. Everything in a non- organic grocery store is inflammatory and has some presence of toxin in it and has had most of the nutrients removed.

h. AVOID NON-ORGANIC MEAT. Ascerone a product containing arsenic that is fed to chickens. The excrement from the chickens is mixed with an unnatural GMO soy and corn fed to the cows in the final 2 months of the cow's life. The cow then puts on 400lbs and gets so toxic that it starts foaming at the mouth. This is the time they slaughter them. The livers are so toxic that they are filled with puss and the stores have stopped making liver available to consumers. On top of injecting them with growth hormones, and anti-biotics they want to radiate the "sick hormone and antibiotic-rich" meat which completely annihilates any food value benefits of Life Force energy to the participant eating it. Bovine growth hormone given animals before slaughter alters your children's development by eating the meat that has been injected. The anti-biotics just keep it alive, by torturing the cow beyond tolerance under normal circumstances.

i. GMO is the elephant in the room. It is not food but a crime against humanity from every scientific report I have read. Genetically Modified food is not food, but "Frankenfood". GMO fed to livestock is killing them dead within 6 months and if the animal lives, leaves them infertile. GMO is currently in your corn, wheat, soy, alphalfa, barley, bran, flour, your ketchup, mayonnaise, and energy boost drinks sold in the pharmacies as a short list. It is in

80% of food products sold in regular grocery stores. When you consume any pastry or bread, anything made from flour that is not organic, notice how the right side of your gut goes into pain and spasm following. The BT corn actually contains pesticides that destroy the stomachs of insects and kills them and harms humans. GMO is not life sustaining but has negative Life force and goes beyond the realm of normal comprehension. GMO is in your baby's formula and something you should familiarize yourself with, and desperately try to keep it out of your body for overall health. I believe that it will take trillions of dollars to clean up, when ethics catch up to humanity waking up. The crops are being burned around the world and are rejected in several countries like France, Hungary and Japan has recently banned any product that might have GMO in it. There are currently 420 million acres around the world growing GMO that need to be burned.

j. MICROWAVES contribute to obesity and weight gain. The microwave rearranges the molecules of your cooked food and water in it to the point where your body doesn't recognize what comes out of it. If you don't believe me, take 2 plants alive in 2 pots. Boil one cup of water on a stove and one cup of water in a microwave. Carefully mark 1 plant to receive water from the microwave and one cup to receive water from the stove after cooling of course and do this daily for 10 days. The plant fed the cooled water from the stove after a week will thrive and the plant fed the cooled water from the microwave will wilt and die, try it for yourself. So anything eaten from a microwave your stomach will look at it as a poison and try and figure out how to get rid of it. Food from this cooking process slows down digestion will cause soft fat obesity, lower energy, and lead to IBS disease. Best to throw in the garbage in case you are tempted to use it.

k. COFFEE kills digestive enzymes, so drink your coffee ½ hour before food or close to 1 hour after eating. Coffee puts your body into a fight or flight situation, restricts blood flow by dilating blood vessels. By definition coffee is a heart attack juice and because coffee is processed, it has no nutritional benefit and it is absent of nutrition and not life sustaining. Coffee is a diuretic which dehydrates you, which concentrates toxins in the body. You need to drink 4 cups of water to replace the diuretic effect of one cup of coffee and it is unhealthy for the liver and an irritant to the stomach of those who drink it.

l. SODA kills digestive enzymes and interferes with nutrient absorption. A cold soda with a burger and fries solidifies the fat in your stomach which contributes to weight gain by slowing the digestive process. The toxins in the liver contributes to obesity as well. Soda contains the most toxic version of HFCS, high fructose corn syrup in food which is the number one cause of cholesterol. Note: organic eggs which are eggs from non-tortured chickens that eat normal diets are good for you and will reduce cholesterol. The less cooked the eggs the better.

m. ALCOHOL kills digestive enzymes, so nutrient absorption is compromised if you consume within a ½ hour of your meal. Alcohol also has the added benefit of wreaking havoc on your liver, pancreas and kidneys. When the liver is not functioning properly you will experience unhealthy weight gain especially in the abdomen. Alcoholics usually go skinny with a pot belly that is a symptom of malnutrition and a toxic liver. Some grow overweight with a pot belly. Nutrient deficiency can reveal itself as overweight for some or skinny legs for others and affects collagen integrity. On a hot day the carbohydrates of a beer in the afternoon at 3pm can help construction workers get to the end of the day with extra energy. Red wine has an anti-oxidant called resveratrol in it, and one glass a day is helpful to reduce inflammation and helps to reduce incidences of heart disease. Resveratrol is found in the skin of red grapes. Headaches from drinking too much alcohol is from dehydration. Drink extra water with electrolytes from a health food store to rehydrate your brain and your body and aloe gel to sooth the irritation of the digestive tract.

n. SMOKING interferes with nutrient absorption by killing digestive enzymes within 1/2 hour of mealtime. I notice that smokers who quit put on 10 lbs. That demonstrates improved nutrient absorption. Caloric intake will dictate the nature of the "weight gain". Healthy diet will yield healthy "weight gain". The best way to quit smoking is reduce stress in your life and follow this chapter from top to bottom. Reducing your stress will increase your pH as well. Increasing your pH is the measure of health and super immunity. I should mention that smoking doesn't cause cancer but contributes to it by weakening the lungs, interferes with nutrient absorption and increases the toxins the liver has to process. By improving your health and raising your pH, addictions and quitting smoking have been proven to be more successful, along with acupuncture in the ear area also improve statistics.

o. MUNICIPAL WATER contributes to obesity where chlorine and fluoride are added to drinking water. These 2 products are as toxic as arsenic, so you are poisoning your poor overworked liver which contributes to obesity. The chlorine or fluoride displaces the iodine from your thyroid and combine that with absence of iodine in your average food intake, and you have your hypothyroidism epidemic in non-rural communities. The biggest culprit is bromine in your hot tub, which is now contained in your breads and cereals that replaced healthy iodine in the manufacturing process. The molecule displaces iodine faster than the other 2 poisons. When Iodine is displaced, the thyroid is deactivated and metabolism just starts to shut down. When your metabolism slows down it doesn't matter how few calories your body consumes, your body will slow down with it. It doesn't matter how much exercise you do with your personal trainer both of you are going to be frustrated with a lack of progress. Sorry. The water is delivered at the tap with no Life Force energy, which is another negative. Your body needs Life Force through what you consume, it is an equation. Water is the blood of the Earth. Life Force of the body's cells start with healthy nourished blood which is fed by what you eat and drink. The skin is the last to receive nutrients from the blood. A town in France uses Oxygen in the municipal water system to deliver water to the tap alive with no poison and at 1/5000th of the chlorine in concentration of North American cities without dissolving the pipes and god knows what those pipes are made of? Oxygen kills disease and delivers water alive at the tap. Your flowers and plants will thrive on it. What your plants and livestock thrive on, people thrive on. Test your plants with water from a pond or bottled water pH 7.0 (natural pH) absent of F (fluoride) on the label and then compare plant growth with water from your municipal supplied tap water and watch the noticeable difference in the way the 3 different water sourced plants thrive. It's interesting to note that 98% of Europe by population doesn't allow fluoride in its drinking water and that most of Europe doesn't allow GMO crops. Most of North America doesn't even know what GMO is, and still thinks mercury dental fillings and fluoride is good for you. Good God Help Us!

p. ANTI BACTERIAL SOAP and household sprays what?? "Anti-bacterial" soap is another name for anti-biotic that kills your probiotics, your good bacteria in your gut, which leads to depression and poor nutrient absorption and obesity, as well as Irritable Bowel Syndrome, raising toxic levels in your liver, weakening the immune system, along with a lowering of your body's pH level in the blood due to inflammation. Anti-bacterial soap, and anti-bacterial sprays etc you see on TV are marketed as slick engineered ergonomic public dispensing stations in hospitals that contribute to obesity. Whatever goes on the skin gets absorbed into the fat and then migrates into the blood stream. This is how hormones are taken, by massaging into the skin. The antibiotic antibacterial soap, and household sprays are absorbed and breathed into the body. The emphasis is on bacteria control but it is the chemicals that are killing us and destroying our immune systems, then creating a problem with bacteria intolerance, where there wasn't a problem before. Oxygen is the healthy answer to soap for any bacteria issues.

q. AVOID the HCG DIET because it requires you to starve yourself of nutrients. Just 500 calories a day, while you burn fat? That is a tremendous amount of stress for temporary results. Any weight loss would be unhealthy and temporary and 500 calories puts you into nutritional deficiency and slows down your metabolism. Again it's not about the calories, weight loss is about your nutritional density. HCG is just a gimmick that doesn't incorporate healthy weight loss using the primary essential elements of health. Avoid any diet or anyone who recommends you going down below 1200 calories a day.

r.   GREEN COFFEE BEAN diet should be avoided. There are more effective ways of reducing fat than the 12 weeks spent on a pill. The green coffee bean contains the drug caffeine that makes you hyper which isn't healthy. No coffee is good for you and because it is in a processed pill form you have a reduction in nutrient value. It is only a single source of nutrient which is an insignificant source of nutrient and if it reduces fat in the liver, it is not an effective means because it is a single source and also processed. Caffeine put tremendous stress on the body, which interferes with normalizing sleep patterns and interferes with allowing your body to be in a calm alert state. This is my opinion, and there are healthier methods to lose weight with your money.

s.   AVOID food that has been processed, cooked, chopped, fried, or cut. Try steaming your vegetables and raw is best for you. Natural food has a higher Life Force energy. Apples have the spin vortex of the earth that gives them its shape of a torus. Apples are best left uncut and eaten whole. The seeds of fruit are an anti-cancerous agent being that of the healthy B17 vitamin Laetrile.

t.   AVOID MEDICATION if you can. Because they are not life sustaining, they are a poison to your body it must get rid of. The poison is collected in the liver where you will begin to see it become inflamed with a consequence of an expanding waist line. They are all inflammatory throughout the body. By removing the symptom of one ailment they stress 10 other functions in your body and have long term consequences causing inflammation and creating cellular scarring over time that is irreversible and leads to dementia, and memory problems associated with old age. Avoid treatment of symptoms and always correct the cause. Medication is just meant to stabilize you until get some real help.

u.   AVOID STATINS!! If you can. Cholesterol is essential along with protein, amino acids and hormones for health. Statins are responsible for too many diseases to list in the weight loss chapter, but one is Alzheimer's disease. By eating organic, juicing, meal replacements, and flushing your organs of toxins and gallstones will eliminate the need for statins with your doctor's approval within weeks.

v. AVOID the LIQUID MEAL or boost replacements sold in pharmacies and non-organic grocery stores. The benefits of their formula are outweighed with negative ingredients that cause inflammation rather than reduce inflammation because of GMO contamination. GMO is the worst culprit found in these formulas that aggravate diabetes and causes inflammation, and organs to begin shutting down along with intestinal damage. Meal replacement formulas in health food stores and on the internet are best. I would avoid meal replacements with soy as an ingredient.

w. AVOID HFCS with high fructose corn syrup, because it is one of the most dangerous source of calories for North Americans. It is a poison that tastes like sugar. Fructose in any form including crystalline fructose is the worst of the worst. Fructose is a refined protein derived from corn, and is used in thousands of food products and drinks. Excessive fructose consumption can cause metabolic damage and triggers the early stages of diabetes and heart disease. It contributes to insulin resistance and heart disease, diabetes, obesity, hypertension, cardiovascular disease, liver disease, cancer, arthritis and more. Fructose is metabolized differently from glucose. The metabolic burden falls on your liver, similar to alcohol resulting in a flood of toxic byproducts. Glucose, on the other hand is your body's nearly ideal source of fuel.

x. AVOID FAT cravings for french fries, potato chips, greasy hamburgers, by taking a double daily dose of EFA (Essential Fatty Acids) that is your omega 3, 6, 9's. By having healthy fats loaded up in your nutrient stores of your body cuts cravings for the bad fats. If you don't believe this to be true, try taking EFA's for a month and then go off it and monitor your cravings for bad fats contained in french fries and potato chips. The EFA's are good for skin, eyes, brain, autism, hair softness, heart, reducing menstrual cramps symptoms over weeks taking it and lowering inflammation in your body. Best to focus on Omega 3's especially to align the imbalance of the bad Omega 6 that is overused as food preservative. This imbalance is a somewhat significant contributor to weight gain. Ratios of Omega 3 to 6 is about 1:15 and it should be naturally 1:3.

y. AVOID SWEETS to avoid sugar spikes followed by hunger cravings. Consume food high in protein with amino acids. Whey proteins eggs, and rice based protein are best. Sugar is the "cocaine addiction" of food. Sweets are low in nutrition and toxic. Sugar feeds cancer and shuts down white blood cell immunity within 20 minutes of digestion. Anything that is not life sustaining is a toxin the body must use valuable Life force energy to get rid of.

z. AVOID STRESS and avoid eating to cope with stress, do an exercise instead like cardio or even better still sex. The love vibration has the lowest stress. Comfort food like Potato Chips alleviates stress. Whatever you put in your shopping cart will end up in your belly. Stress is actually reduced by raising pH of your blood. Lack of sleep or poor quality sleep contributes to being overweight. Cortisol rises when you are stressed which can lead to packing weight around the middle. It's best to let stress pass through you and not to hold it. Find a way around a traffic jam and stop for a salad. Get healthy and experience more love in your life. People who can't handle stress have the lowest frequency and it is a symptom of poor health, low pH and a toxic gut of improper ratios corrected by probiotics over time. Your thoughts don't cause disease but your ability to diffuse stress will help you, every minute a negative thought comes up that causes stress or anxiety consciously let it go. Fear is "False Evidence Appearing Real", and is thought of as the lowest vibration. Fear is rammed down your throat your entire life. Try thinking of something good in your life from the past, present or the future and stay there. Stress is ok everyone experiences stress and stressful thoughts, it's just how you deal with them that matter. Gratitude is the best attitude. Appreciate your lessons.

zz. AVOID WHEAT, Complex whole wheat and grains raises blood sugar more effectively than sugar itself and triggers resistance to insulin, and visceral fat. Wheat is perfect for contributing to obesity, IBS, and lowering the celiac threshold of intolerance for autoimmune patients exposed to mold. Wheat gliadin protein is an appetite stimulant, and is added to salad dressings, soups, prepared food, frozen food and just about every food in a grocery store, even licorice. Another reason to avoid non-organic food in regular grocery stores.

There are several layers to being fat or obese. Each layer you address reduces unhealthy fat and contributes to healthy muscle. All relate back to what your body needs and doesn't need. The cure for obesity is to focus on lowering your inflammation. Eliminating inflammation is the key to super immunity, thriving and finding ideal weight. Losing weight does not achieve health because it has ignored the cause of weight gain. Avoid stress, find passion, love and harmony through health. Cleanse and flush your liver and kidneys as you would your car's filters, and consume non-toxic hydrating fluids and eat unprocessed organic food that has a high density of nutrition contained. Add a few supplements and meal replacement daily, best from a health food store and not a department or grocery store and take hormones best by prescription from a specialist MD after age 40. Discover juiced organic vegetables and fruit. Stay away from breathing toxic environmental mold in your home, your place of work or where you vacation especially by the ocean. Warm moist air and central air conditioners that don't drain water properly are sources of autoimmune disease. This is as simple as I can put it, all have an impact on excess weight. Diet and exercise can hurt you and delay, distract and detract you from the truth.

Warning: Pharmaceuticals are getting in the game of weight loss now. They are suggesting that obesity is a disease but it is not. It is merely a symptom of inflammation. The principal of treating obesity with poison is absurd and can only harm you. 97% of pharmaceutical drugs are obsolete, dangerous and should be taken temporarily until you get yourself back to health. Be warned that your government is not working on your behalf. Baby formula sold in the aisles of grocery stores and pharmacies now has estrogen mimickers that are 100x stronger than birth control pills and GMO contained that mutate cell development of your child. Some babies are responding to unbalanced hormones by becoming obese and the doctor's recommendation was bariatric surgery for a 2 year as a solution last week!

Tips:

When your body feels pain that is its signal that something is wrong. When your body is tired listen to it and get some sleep. If you wake up feeling exhausted, yet had good uninterrupted sleep you probably have toxic mold in your room or house where you sleep. Being in mold can have an incredible effect on making you feel exhausted proportional to the intensity of the contamination.

I believe that the strict limits set for organic is too high. I believe there should be 2 levels of classification. The most important minimum precedent be that the nutrition is in tact in what you are eating, where the soil is pesticide free, managed and crops rotated. Costs for organic produce can then come down. Many foods are organic but are not labeled as such and this is a tragedy to the growers and the consumers who need a fresh reliable supply!!

FRESH FOOD is a distraction because it is not indicative of healthy food. Think of it as fresh nutrient deficient and toxin enriched from now on, or be suspect of this. It needs to be mentioned because this type of food tastes good but will cause weight gain and disease. Chicken nuggets contain TBHQ which is tertiary butylhydroquinone, which is a form of butane derived from petroleum. It can keep food "fresh" for years, some 14 years of the pictures I have seen. Consuming a single gram of TBHQ causes suffocation, vomiting and collapse. Food that contains this ingredient is not food nor is it life sustaining. TBHQ has a serious negative Life Force energy that puts your body into inflammation which over time leads to obesity, disease and in concentration, death.

There are 75,000 chemicals, which are poisons in the food chain, and a baby starts out on average with 200 chemicals found in the umbilical cord. These chemicals are poisonous because they are not life sustaining. I don't think any are necessary and there needs to be a law that bans chemicals and toxins from food and water. Exceptions can be made, but decisions are preferred by ethical people with common sense with moral ethics please.

Raspberry natural flavor comes from the anal sac of a beaver. All artificial raspberry flavored food products like ice cream, yogurt, teas, candies, jell-o, fruit flavored drinks contain it as a key component.

Milk contains estrogen 100,000x more toxic than estrogen found in pesticides. Consumption of natural estrogen contained in milk and cheese leads to breast cancer, ovarian cancer and testicular cancer among men aged 20-39, and is a major cause of acne.

Antifreeze or propylene glycol is used in cars to prevent freezing of your radiator. The chemical is extremely toxic and is used in commercial ice cream to prevent it from getting frozen hard.

The artificial vanilla flavored food products like soda, candy, yogurts and baked cookies comes from a waste product of the wood pulp industries.

Try to avoid food that contains more than 6 ingredients as a rule of thumb to use when looking at labels. The ingredients you should recognize from your kitchen shelves and not something from a laboratory.

While you are at work the FDA (Food and Drug Administration) is allowing toxic substances to be added to every product in a grocery store and is overseeing the systematic elimination of nutrients with their approval, "for your safety"? It might be a good time to switch your purchases to organic and let this stuff rot on the shelves, if it has an expiry date? Be aware of agendas that employ phrases like, "for your safety" or "natural" or "healthy", they generally mean the opposite. The psychopaths are running the insane asylum, and business is good.

It has been proven already by ethical science that organic fruits and vegetables grown without pesticides in the soil are vastly superior. Most science now is unethical where scientists are bought and paid for by corporations to report information contrary to scientific results. The silence of politicians to this fraud is consent and therefore collusion. Who do you think said smoking was good for you, and there is example after example over my research of misleading advertising to the point of it being criminal fraud hurting a massive amount of people. Over 90% of scientists graduating from University are using their talents employed by industry to come up with more and more chemicals to flavor, induce addictions, preserve and color our food and drink which promotes death and look the other way. I've noticed that, the slicker the packaging and the cartoon characters, the better the aroma, the cheaper the food, the more likely it is to have had the nutrients removed and toxins loaded up. Executives of these corporations and the scientists using their talents, that are knowingly hurting people on a massive scale have a fiduciary duty to come forward now or be thrown in jail. I think life sentences would fit the crime.

I had a friend who went off meal replacements, juicing, cleansing and went back to regular food and started to get fat around the middle. He told me meal replacement and cleansing didn't work because he got fat again. This was a thought from an intelligent successful businessman with high intelligence. When you go off healthy food and cleansing, your body will go back into inflammation. If you know your body lives off nutrients, why not meet that need for life?

Profound results with profound effort is required for anyone who has disease, or any athlete trying to improve their health, or anyone trying to lose weight, or anyone who just wants to thrive.

Common Sense is like deodorant, those that need it most don't use it.

To the readers and all,

I am not authorized to advise or help anyone on how to treat disease or give recommendations about health. Ideas in this book are just points to consider on your path to wellness and enlightenment. This is my story and everyone's recovery can be different in their responses to the protocols I used for myself. The subject matter is for discussion purposes only for helping humanity realize that health care in the developed world does not exist and a new future going forward still needs to embrace the idea of treating the cause of disease and not the symptoms. When the realization that nutrition gives life and that toxins kill life, a concept society and the medical community hasn't quite realized yet, suffering of humanity can begin to subside. Many successes discussed have not been FDA assessed or peer reviewed. My belief is that this is our future of health, ideas of which are much different than the current standard. The ideas don't need to make sense now but will plant a seed for later. The law states that only your doctor can treat any medical condition or disease. Until you experience, you won't understand why. Choosing wisely is a personal choice you must make for yourself!

Answer from chapter 1:

Open the refrigerator and put the penguin in and close the door. This tests whether you tend to do simple things in a complicated way....Continued chap 3.

Chapter 3

Toxic blood = Autoimmune = Biotoxin Illness

Toxic Blood is the number one cause of disease and inflammation, so it is the most important element in the Matrix when diagnosing any patient of illness. There is a doctor in the US that has a protocol your laymen would call a cure sitting on his desk with a success rate of 100% on 10,000 patients collecting dust for over 15 years. His accuracy at assessing this disease, diagnosing and confirming symptoms, using DNA and blood tests, while explaining the science of how the disease works for all 170 autoimmune listed is extraordinary. It is the most brilliant and successful work ever conducted in the history of health care. The cure for autoimmune disease under current regulations is unable to share, and as a consequence millions are suffering and a few are profiting from policy instead of common sense.

Autoimmune isn't about your body attacking itself, but is a neurological disease that manifests itself physically in 170 different ways. It is not an autoimmune disease because you don't have an autoimmune system. It is an innate immune system response to neurotoxins in the blood called a cytokine storm that recirculates itself to cause chronic fatigue in all autoimmune patients. I have profound knowledge as a patient on the subject of autoimmune after suffering with it for 36 years and finding the doctor that rid me of this horrible disease that enabled me to get out my wheelchair in short order after being immobile for close to 2 years. He was the doctor who put an end to 36 years of suffering.

I had discovered the other 4 elements of the Matrix and together with the doctor's protocol, got me free of my wheelchair. I was free at last!! Autoimmune was the key to unlocking the Matrix of health which was the most important element and the most evasive because without the doctor's cure I would still be in my wheelchair. It is the one element of the 5 that causes the worst inflammation and has the most impact on pH and trumps the other 4 less significant elements utterly and completely proportional to intensity of toxic mold exposure or neurotoxins over time. There isn't a healer or a doctor I met who understands autoimmune and that currently leaves all doctors and healers chasing their tails. That is about to change.

The cure for auto immune was found in 1998 by accident. He is not allowed to speak on the subject, I don't have his authorization, and he is not allowed to treat or diagnose anyone with this disease. We need to get support quickly for him and his protocol because he is approaching retirement age. When he does, the Authority has won and the people have lost. There are patients around the world having their intestines cut out today that don't need to if they could only get help from this doctor. The cure for people with autoimmune disease is at your local drug store and your doctor and your rheumatologist doesn't know how to dose it and are not allowed to prescribe it, and don't know what they are, and to my surprise don't care and aren't even curious. I've met enough of them to know. Dogs just chasing their tails with egos so entrenched, it's spectacular to observe when I try and tell them of 100% success and the doctor they should be following!

For Autoimmune:

1 Remove yourself from source of neurotoxins (mold +99% of all cases)

2 Remove cause of inflammation and some pain (cytokines C3a, C4a)

3 Remove major cause of pain (re-regulate transforming growth factor TGF-b1 in blood) or: Go on a non-amylose diet to lower VEGF (

4 Mitigate inflammation and major pain (Vaso Intestinal Peptide)

Autoimmune has the biggest impact on destroying health for several different reasons but one of the worst reasons is that it stops your body's ability to heal itself. Leaky gut does not cause autoimmune but aggravates it with infection. Leaky gut is associated with autoimmune as a symptom because of persistent irritation with the presence of neurotoxins in the blood from mold that can focus on the digestive tract, perhaps because of gene weakness or because of normal function of digesting toxic food and GMO's that are irritating.

It won't matter if you have a great diet all organic, your liver cleansed, have a great life of low stress and work, exercise regularly, take bio available hormones and are surrounded by abundance. If you have a flood in your basement or move into a residence that has significant mold in it, your exposure to toxic mold will have your blood pH crash along with your immune system, your energy, and with your inflammation climbing and you won't be well. You won't respond to antibiotics well and you will bewilder your doctors with your symptoms because in their training they assume you are not in mold and if you assume you are in mold where you live and work, 99% of the mold tested using air samples don't work because of the false negatives. What is worse than no test for mold is a test that is a false negative. The path of your health can deteriorate into a 1000 different directions from exposure, so it is hard to figure out and with no standard for testing, no treatment or diagnosis in North America or the world currently for autoimmune disease, it is one of society's biggest liabilities there is in the community. It seems almost every negative symptom you experience you should start diagnosis assuming that illness could have come from exposure to mold and start from there, especially if illness is recurring. I can think of kids off school regularly, toothaches, colds, flu, and illness associated with a poor immune system. It is a prime suspect for those who are sick regularly from mold and most don't know it.

Mold gives off a toxic gas that permeates throughout a home or workplace but there are many other organisms in our environment that are known to produce biotoxins, like Red tide that floats on the ocean off Vancouver Island Canada and off Sarasota Florida in warm water seasons and also but rarely from the bite of the brown recluse spider. Once this disruptive cycle of exposure to mold continues long enough, it often results in disabling fatigue, problems thinking or remembering things, lack of motivation, depression, problems sleeping, mood changes, neurological symptoms, digestive problems and a list of other symptoms due to biotoxin or neurotoxin exposure. Because each person is biochemically unique, the symptoms of autoimmune can be different for each person. Until now, this had made diagnosis difficult. Biotoxin stands for biological in source and toxic in nature.

The doctor has cured 10,000 people of autoimmune disease with 100% success. 92% of his patients recovered 75% of symptoms within 30 days and the remaining 8% of those who were most severe within 6 to 12 months. The ratio is changing with the most severe increasing perhaps from deteriorating economic conditions and the flawed building code using a plastic vapor barrier with contaminated air fostering more incidences of mold growth in homes. The FDA has been breathing down the doctor's neck analyzing his every move since 1998 when he came forth with his discovery. The FDA does not want this cure out for autoimmune or chronic lyme, nor the cure for MS which are all related to neurotoxins attacking tissue in the body. For MS, it is the myelin sheath tissue that dissolves from the innate immune system response. Another problem is that there is no law that insists that a cure for a disease be used to help patients in North America, the FDA and related agencies makes the laws and enforces them. I found the laws they make are arbitrary to suit corporate interests and not that of patient well-being. The only thing more outrageous than a dumb law is someone who enforces it. His protocol which I will try to explain as best I can is the only one that can cure autoimmune disease or Biotoxin Illness as it will be referred to in the future when it is allowed to come forth. Cure means profound improvement in health by laymen standards. Bentonite clay supplement from a health food store taken by tablespoon daily on an empty stomach helps with autoimmune symptoms until access to treatment can become available. The doctor has been given a research grant to stop treating patients and go do more research. I think it is an inexpensive ploy to have him "go away".

Mold Exposure

To compound the problem of autoimmune, 35% of homes in North America cause symptoms of autoimmune/biotoxin illness due to flawed building codes that put residents to live in plastic bags with steep temperature gradients indoors, to the temperatures that exist outside of their homes. One little prick in your plastic vapor barrier, perhaps a nail for a picture or mirror, or the building inspector misses a nail sized hole opening in a fold of plastic in a corner and you have contamination of warm moist air hitting the cold area of the insulation to have a garden of toxic mold behind the wall. That small contamination is then the breeding ground for a poisonous gas off of mold that permeates throughout the house. Mold is not about the spores, so measurement of them is of no use. Another concern is that particle board seems to have an accelerator agent in it that promotes toxic mold growth that is commonly used in the construction of homes. Carpet and broadloom are just petri dishes for mold. When the carpets are new they gas off toxins and as they age they become toxic mold centers.

About 40% of North Americans are suffering from autoimmune symptoms and it is these symptoms that are confusing doctors, because autoimmune is a multi-symptom, multi-system disease unique to each individual. There are 80 symptoms to autoimmune, 40 are most prevalent and please know that only autoimmune disease can deform and damage the body internally and externally as a consequence of prolonged innate immune system response.

There are blood tests for autoimmune/biotoxin illness that cost 3000$ for a full blood panel with DNA test performed, but abbreviated tests for just C3a and C4a blood test should be enough or an ERMI (environmental rating mold index from that measures from 1 to 4) test for mold done by www.mycometrics.com out of NJ, that costs 300US$.

Toxic Blood Maps the Body for Inflammation

Anything you were born with you will leave the world with. Any change in health that you weren't born with is a consequence of your environment and what you picked up during life. Break down in health will be a result of a gene weakness and/or the consequences of neglect of your body's needs like rest, adequate nutrition, avoiding excessive alcohol, low stress and blood absent of neurotoxins. These can all aggravate inflammation in your body especially when neurotoxins from exposure to mold come and goes. When mold comes alive it can drop you with migraines and or profound fatigue. It comes and goes with the seasons and between rain cycles after reaching perfect levels of humidity along with temperature. It is best to run a dehumidifier in your basement around the clock to avoid perfect conditions for mold. Most people don't know and refuse to accept that their house has mold in it, and that can make those who live in them sick. Each member will respond with different symptoms and severity living in a sick house. The clues are subtle but they are there and escalate and pulsate in regards to symptoms between blooms. You cannot be allergic to mold. It is like saying you are allergic to poison.

Your health is like the water level in an aquarium. When the water level falls in your aquarium it exposes the rocks of disease just below the surface about to erupt with just a trigger, caused perhaps with gene weakness and any of life's neglect. A weak gene or an abused kidney or liver of a heavy drinker or someone with IBS is just waiting to be exposed and it is done through blood flow to inflamed areas of your body. Weak genes just open up potholes of susceptibility.

When you fire a muscle to work there are 2 types of inflammation over time. One is from a lack of nutrients in the blood to repair the worked muscle resulting in inflammation, and the second is where repair is needed but there is a presence of neurotoxins and damage is accelerated. When a muscle is used there is a small amount of inflammation of the muscle after use and that inflammation is intensified with increased blood flow that attracts neurotoxins present in the blood. When neurotoxins are present, they are tagged by the innate immune system that takes out the neurotoxin as it should, but along with it a small sample of tissue, bone, cartilage goes with it from the inflamed area. People with autoimmune shouldn't be exercising because you are actually destroying the muscles most used in your body over time. With autoimmune, your ability to repair itself is compromised proportionately to the level of neurotoxins in the blood. That is why knee and hip replacement along with arthritis in the hands is prevalent. 24% of the population have the gene for autoimmune on chromosome 6 of the innate immune system, that reabsorb the neurotoxin over and over as a result. All autoimmune patients will experience chronic fatigue, so you will have a lot of energy to look forward to once mold and symptoms are eliminated.

40 common Autoimmune/ Biotoxin Illness Symptoms:

- Exhaustion
- Weakness
- Aches
- Cramps
- Unusual pain
- Ice pick pain
- Head ache
- Light sensitivity
- Red eyes
- Blurred
- Tearing
- Sinus
- Cough
- Shortness of breath
- Abdominal pain
- Diarrhea
- Joint Pain
- Morning stiffness
- Memory problems
- Lack of focus/ concentration
- Poor word recall
- Decreased assimilation of new knowledge
- Confusion
- Disorientation
- Skin sensitivity
- Mood swings
- Appetite changes
- Cold sweats
- Poor temperature regulation
- Thirst
- Increased urination
- Static shocks
- Numbness
- Tingling
- Vertigo
- Metallic taste
- Asthma
- ADHD/ADD (contributes)
- Depression
- Apathy/ laziness

Diagnostic Blood Lab below:

HLA-dr is human leukocyte antigens which is done on Chromosome 6 for all patients. It is used by doctors for liver transplants to predict organ rejection and knowledge of this gene mapping technique is rare to doctors. 52b is a common subtype of autoimmune patients. Chromosome 6 refers to the "innate immune" system gene.

MSH (alpha Melanocyte Stimulating Hormone) falls off from the presence of inflammation from autoimmune. The lack of it makes you depressed from low endorphins and increases your sensitivity to pain and increases your susceptibility to sunburn. MSH is available but not permitted to be sold to the public by the system. It is the most essential element for recovery by all auto immune patients and MSH restoration to normal levels is helped by VIP (vaso intestinal peptides) by prescription spayed in the nose

4x/day kept in a refrigerator. VIP is shipped on ice out of a compounding pharmacy in Hopkinton MA in the US.

C3a Immune response

C4a When elevated, both trigger cytokine innate immune response. The body's other immune system is the adaptive immune system that responds to invaders of bacteria and virus related to colds and flu. Vaccinations are that more dangerous because they bypass the adaptive immune response.

TGF-b1 (Transforming Growth Factor) in autoimmune patients is one of the biggest sources of pain to your body. I reduced these levels with one prescription of Cozaar once-a-day from a local pharmacy for 15 days, where I no longer found any benefit I stopped taking it. Cozaar is hard on the kidneys and I drank parsley tea made from organic parsley for a week following to reduce pain in my kidneys. TGF is a protein that controls proliferation, cellular differentiation, and other functions in most cells. It is a type of cytokine which plays a role in immunity, cancer, bronchial asthma, heart disease, diabetes and autoimmune. Cozaar was my friend to effectively reduce pain in my body and so was a mug or 2/day of parsley tea for my kidneys following.

TNF-b1 Tumor Necrosis Factor was a major source of pain I managed to lower by taking the Larch tree extract supplement the medical community is unaware of but I believe the FDA is. The supplement only costs 15$ and is substantially beneficial to all patients for autoimmune and cancer treatment. I used Larch to aid my body to eliminate cancer and it helped with symptoms of pain for autoimmune (see Cancer chapter 8). Larch lowered pain at the source and was not a pill to temporarily interrupt pain.

Western Blot Lyme test is not done in Canada and costs about 400$ in the US and is about 50% accurate. The Canadian test is about 5% accurate called the ELISA test (Enzyme-linked immunosorbent assay). Perhaps this test is used because someone's relative owns the lab? For Chronic Lyme it is actually more difficult to treat than autoimmune by itself because you have kill the spirochete parasites first and then deal with autoimmune following from the toxic die off. 24% who are susceptible to Chronic

Lyme of 100% who contract Lyme disease. There is a DNA test that confirms susceptibility for chronic Lyme and autoimmune. The medical community currently is trying to avoid acknowledgement of the disease and a few doctors use an archaic form of antibiotics for months up to 24 to treat the parasites of Lyme. More efficient methods to kill bacteria using MMS, h2o2, ozone, or Rife frequency which matches the frequency of the spirochete to blow it up using resonance. All have been proven to work with superior results without consequences of giving up the health of your gut from taking antibiotics. You have to be cautious of the rate of toxic die-off of the parasite in your blood because it causes toxic shock and the symptoms begin with headaches, fatigue, a fever and nausea that can escalate to be severe. Killing the parasite needs to be paced according to tolerance of your body's ability to eliminate. It is caused from the bite of a tick found in nature and can be at your picnics. Most are not contaminated and they are spreading by attaching to birds and animals. Lyme and a lot of "unnatural" biological diseases and irregularities world-wide are thought to come from Plum Island off the coast of Lyme Connecticut where 100's of scientists are doing biological warfare research full time. It is rumored they are planning to move this lab west because of a lot questions being asked by Americans recently.

Below are the tests for autoimmune that measure for DNA, inflammation responses, and hormones irregularities. Hormones are sent out of normal range with inflammatory response of the innate immune system due to the presence of neurotoxins from exposure to toxic mold in your environment you breathe. Leptin is one of the hormone responses that when raised, triggers obesity.

Blood Test for Autoimmune or Biotoxin Illness

Blood Draw	Normal Range
HLA (RS)	N/A
MSH	35-81 pg/mL
Leptin	Male 0.5-13.8 ng/mL female1.1-27.5
ADH	1.0-13.3 pg/ml

Osmo	280-300 mosmol
ACTH	9-52 pg/mL
Cortisol	**am** 4.3-22.4 / **pm** 3.1-16.7 ug/dL
DHEAS	Male 59-452 ug/dL female 76-255
Testosterone	Male 241-827 ng/dL female 20-55 pre 7-40 post
Androstenedione	Male 50-250 ng/dL female **47-268** ng/dL
CRP	0.0-4.9 mg/L
ESR	0-30
TNF	<8 pg/mL
IL-1B	0.00-3.73 pg/mL
IL 6	
IL 10	
Alpha Interferon	
Beta Interferon	
Gamma Interferon	
MMP-9	85-332 ng/mL
PAI-1	2-14 IU/mL
Lipid Pheno (RS)	N/A
CBC	N/A
CMP	N/A
GGT	0-65 IU/L
Nasal Culture (RS)	
VEGF	31-86 pg/mL
Erythropoietin	9.0-19.5 mU/mL
Anticardiolipins (RS)	**IgA** 0-12, **IgG** 0-10, **IgM** 0-9
Myelin Basic Protein EIA	units <8
AGA, IgA, IgG (RS)	0-19
C2	1.6-3.5 mg/dl
C3	90-180 mg/dl
C4	16-47 mg/dl
C1q-IC	<4.4 ug Eq/ml
C3d-IC	<24 ug/ml

C4d	0.9-8.0 mg/dl
Prop B	12-53 mg/dl
C3a	<146 ng/ml
IgE	0-158 IU/mL
Lyme Western Blot (RS)	
TSH	0.3-5.0 uIU/mL
Ubiquinone	

Neurotoxin presence in the blood from exposure to toxic mold can be measured by a C3a and C4a cytokine immune response in the blood by a test. Mold can be intense periodically and usually comes in waves every couple of weeks or once a month. Its intensity increases during the winter and periods, when the sun isn't shining, and the weather is damp and cold. This type of home or work environment can put you into a wheelchair or under the knife over time. I found that profoundly moldy places have constant toxic levels that can make you chronically sick with severity. I've been in a home like this where a death had occurred, and there was evidence of severe mold with plastic tarps on the ceiling with pools of water in them. The cause of death was a ruptured spleen and I knew that wasn't the cause of death but was only a symptom. The death was from complications from toxic mold exposure that could have been confirmed by a blood test not available in Canada. Mold is a poisonous gas that leaves its thumb print in dust collected behind the fridge and in carpet where dust particles later are prepared for the petri dish for mold to grow in the lab by microbiologists to observe and report. This is an example of ethical science working with certainty and efficiency.

For 100% of all autoimmune patients, cholestyramine is the protocol for 15 to 30 days. Cholestyramine or Olestyr is not a drug but is dispensed by prescription at your local drug store. Good luck trying to get that medication from your doctor. It seems they are not compensated for prescribing it and/or they are not allowed to dispense it for autoimmune. The FDA (Food and Drug Administration) has known that it corrects symptoms of autoimmune by removing neurotoxins out of the blood since the 1990's once the patient is out of mold is when it is effective. It is meant to lower cholesterol but binds with neurotoxins in the bile duct of the liver without any chemical interaction with your body's chemistry. Its only function is as a binder for excretion that just passes through the body. 92% of patients were cured 75% of symptoms within 30 days for autoimmune, once out of mold, on a sample of patients approaching 10,000. The balance of the 8% took 6-12 months to eliminate symptoms of autoimmune once out of mold with more elaborate treatment.

One of the 10 treatments involves switching to a non-amylose diet with an Rx of Actose for 10-15 days. The no amylase diet is to eliminate foods that contain a high concentration of amylose, a complex carbohydrate found in wheat and cereal grains. They contain high amounts of this carbohydrate along with food grown in the ground except onion and garlic. Actose is a drug meant for diabetics but it can be used to manipulate cell communication as a requirement for recovery for some patients depending on DNA and blood lab results. Note: I think Olestyr was replaced with statin drugs to lower cholesterol, because the Authorities realized it was also curing autoimmune patients. The substitute with statin drugs are dangerous to your health and lead to a multitude of diseases, because cholesterol is an essential element to the building blocks of cellular life.

These diseases are only symptoms of autoimmune/Biotoxin Illness. If you go on Wikipedia, you can see how each of them deforms a part of your anatomy and lucky for you if you have been diagnosed with something on the list below, because there is a solution for each and every one of you. The list of diseases are 170 symptoms of biotoxin illness or autoimmune disease that have the same cause, manifesting itself according to one's DNA. Chronic fatigue is the one thing all have in common. The disease does not come from your head but from your body and causes depression and brain fog and a host of chronic physical limitations to life.

Autoimmune/biotoxin diseases listed:

You will notice how everyone listed has some kind of degenerative impact on the body.

Acute disseminated encephalomyelitis - Disease of the brain following vaccination/infection
Addison's disease - Adrenal / Endocrine disorder
Agammaglobulinemia - Immune deficiency

Alopecia Areata - Irregular hair loss

Amyotrophic Lateral Sclerosis - Lu Gerhrigs

Ankylosing Spondylitis - Inflammation of the skeleton and joints

Anti Phospholipid Syndrome - provokes blood clots (thrombosis) in both arteries / veins

Antisynthetase syndrome - rare medical syndrome associated with Interstitial lung disease, dermatomyositis

Atopic allergy - Immunal Globulin E reaction to Allergen

Atopic dermatitis - Like Eczema

aplastic anemia - Bone Marrow disease damages formation of blood cells

Autoimmune cardiomyopathy - heart becomes weakened, enlarged and cannot pump blood efficiently

Autoimmune enteropathy - is a rare cause of intractable diarrhea associated with circulating gut autoantibodies

Autoimmune hemolytic anemia - occurs when antibodies directed against the person's own red blood cells

Autoimmune hepatitis - disease of the liver that occurs when the body's immune system attacks cells of the liver

Autoimmune inner ear disease - rapid progressive bilateral sensorineural hearing loss

Autoimmune lymphoproliferative syndrome - Accumulation of excess lymphocytes results in enlargement of the lymph nodes, the liver, and the spleen

Autoimmune peripheral neuropathy - causes diabetes, shingles, vitamin deficiency

Autoimmune pancreatitis - primary inflammatory sclerosis of the pancreas

Autoimmune polyendocrine syndrome

Autoimmune progesterone dermatitis-correspond 2 progesterone levels during menstrual cycle

Autoimmune thrombocytopenic purpura - low platelet count with normal bone marrow

Autoimmune uveitis - Severe inflammation of the eye

Balo concentric sclerosis - Similar to Multiple sclerosis

Behçet's disease - mucous membrane ulceration and ocular problems

Berger's disease IgA *Nephropathy* means damage to or disease of a kidney. IgA represents 75% of your body's immune system.

Bickerstaff's encephalitis - inflammatory disorder of the central nervous system

Blau syndrome - similar to sarcoidosis and granuloma annulare

Bullous pemphigoid - blisters at the space between skin layers epidermis and dermis

Cancer - cells divide and grow uncontrollably. Most cancer stems from autoimmune

Castleman's disease - may develop in the lymph node tissue at a single site or throughout the body

Celiac disease - pain and discomfort in the digestive tract small intestine

Chagas disease - tropical parasitic disease

Chronic Fatigue - is a symptom of all autoimmune patients

Chronic inflammatory demyelinating polyneuropathy - immune-mediated inflammatory disorder of the peripheral nervous system

Chronic Lymes is the symptom following Lymes disease, where the toxins from the die off of the spirochetes begins an autoimmune reaction that takes you from the frying pan and puts you into the fire.

Chronic recurrent multifocal osteomyelitis - bones have lesions, inflammation, and pain

Chronic obstructive pulmonary disease - airways narrow over time (copd)

Churg-Strauss syndrome - airway inflammation

Cicatricial pemphigoid - skin lesions of the mucous membranes and skin

Cogan syndrome - recurrent inflammation of the front of the eye (the cornea)

Cold agglutinin disease - high IgM, directed against red blood cells

Complement component 2 deficiency - is a protein that in humans is encoded by the *C2* gene

Contact dermatitis - localized rash or irritation of the skin

Cranial arteritis - is a form of vasculitis of the head

CREST syndrome - a connective tissue disease

Crohn's disease - chronic inflammatory disorder of gastrointestinal tract

Cushing's Syndrome - excess cortisol

Cutaneous leukocytoclastic angiitis - inflammation of small blood vessels

Dego's disease - affects the lining of the medium and small veins and arteries

Dercum's disease - nervous system dysfunction, mechanical pressure on nerve

Dermatitis herpetiformis - chronic blistering skin condition

Dermatomyositis - inflammation of the muscles and the skin

Diabetes mellitus type 1 - destruction of insulin-producing beta cells of the pancreas

Diffuse cutaneous sclerosis - thickening of the skin caused by accumulation of collagen

Dressler's syndrome - the outer lining of the heart

Drug-induced lupus - drugs cause an autoimmune response

Discoid lupus erythematosus - chronic skin condition of sores

Eczema - recurring skin rashes, redness, swelling, dry crusting, itchy

Endometriosis - inflammation of the female reproductive organ

Enthesitis - inflammation where tendons or ligaments insert into the bone

Eosinophilic fasciitis - diseases that affect the connective tissues surrounding muscles

Eosinophilic gastroenteritis - damage to the gastrointestinal tract wall

Eosinophilic pneumonia - white blood cell called an eosinophil accumulates in the lung

Epidermolysis bullosa acquisita - chronic subepidermal blistering of the skin

Erythema nodosum - inflammation of the fat cells under the skin

Erythroblastosis - antibodies are some which attack the red blood cells of the newborn

Essential mixed cryoglobulinemia - blood contains large amounts of insoluable Immunoglobulins

Evan's syndrome - antibodies attack their own red blood cells and platelets

Fibrodysplasia ossificans progressive - damaged soft tissue regrows as bone

Gastritis - inflammation of the lining of the stomach

Glomerulonephritis - renal diseases usually affecting both kidneys

Goodpasture's syndrome - antibodies attack the lungs and kidneys, leading to bleeding

Graves' disease - commonly affects the thyroid, causes hyperthyroidism, goiters

Guillain-Barré syndrome - disorder affecting the peripheral nervous system

Hashimoto's encephalopathy - hypothyroidism stroke-like symptoms confirmed by elevated anti-thyroid antibodies

Hashimoto's thyroiditis - most common cause of primary hypothyroidism, false iodine is.

Henoch-Schonlein purpura - disease of skin, other organs that mostly affects children

Herpes gestationis - blistering skin disease that occurs during pregnancy, not herpes virus

Hidradenitis suppurativa - skin disease that affects areas bearing apocrine sweat glands

Hughes-Stovin syndrome - pulmonary artery aneurysms and deep vein thrombosis

Hypogammaglobulinemia - immune deficiency reduction of gamma globulins

Idiopathic inflammatory demyelinating diseases - a variant of multiple sclerosis

Idiopathic pulmonary fibrosis - fibrosis of the supporting framework of the lung a chronic progressive form of lung disease

Idiopathic thrombocytopenic purpura - is defined as isolated low platelet count

IgA nephropathy - inflammation of the kidney

Inclusion body myositis - weakness and wasting of both distal and proximal muscles

Chronic inflammatory demyelinating polyneuropathy - immune-mediated inflammatory disorder of the peripheral nervous system

Interstitial cystitis - bladder pain associated with urinary urgency and frequency

Juvenile rheumatoid arthritis - caused by vaccinations, reaction to squaline

Kawasaki's disease - blood vessels throughout the body become inflamed

Lambert-Eaton myasthenic syndrome - disorder that is characterised by muscle weakness of the limbs

Leukocytoclastic vasculitis - inflammation of small blood vessels

Lichen planus - disease that affects the skin, tongue, and oral mucosa

Lichen sclerosus - white skin patches, may cause scarring on and around genital area

Linear IgA disease - blistering disease

Lupoid hepatitis - causes liver cirrhosis

Lupus erythematosus - immune system becomes hyperactive and attacks healthy tissues

Majeed syndrome - skin disorder

Ménière's disease - disorder of the inner ear that can affect hearing and balance

Microscopic polyangiitis - symptoms of fever, anorexia, weight loss, fatigue, renal failure

Miller-Fisher syndrome - similar to Guillain–Barré syndrome

Morphea - connective tissue disease

Mucha-Habermann disease - can cause ulcers on the exterior, looks like chicken pox

Multiple sclerosis - insulating covers of nerve cells in the brain, spinal cord are damaged

Myasthenia gravis - fluctuating muscle weakness, sometimes in the eye

Myositis - inflammation of the muscle from lipid-lowering drugs statins

Narcolepsy - brain's inability to regulate sleep-wake cycles

Neuromyelitis optica - inflammation and demyelination of the optic nerve

Neuromyotonia - hyperexcitability that causes spontaneous muscular activity

Occular cicatricial pemphigoid - erosive skin lesions of mucous membranes and skin

Opsoclonus myoclonus syndrome - rare neurological disorder

Ord's thyroiditis - body's own antibodies fight the cells of the thyroid

Palindromic Rheumatism - acute pain, redness, swelling, of one, usually or multiple joints

Pandas pediatric autoimmune neuropsychiatric disorders associated with streptococcus

Paraneoplastic cerebellar degeneration - reaction targeted against components of the central nervous system

Paroxysmal nocturnal hemoglobinuria - anemia due to destruction of red blood cells

Parry Romberg syndrome - degeneration of the tissues beneath the skin

Parsonage-Turner syndrome - sudden pain radiating from the shoulder to the upper arm

Pars planitis - inflammation of the eye, can be serious

Pemphigus vulgaris - blistering skin disease with skin lesions

Pernicious anaemia - leads to vitamin B_{12} deficiency

Poems syndrome - Myeloma is the most common plasma cell proliferation

Polyarteritis nodosa - affects arteries, the blood vessels

Polymyalgia rheumatica - pain in many muscles

Polymyositis - chronic inflammation of the muscles

Primary biliary cirrhosis - progressive destruction of the small bile ducts of the liver

Primary sclerosing cholangitis - disease of the bile ducts

Primary biliary cirrhosis - destruction of the small bile ducts of the liver

Progressive inflammatory neuropathy - paralysis, pain, fatigue, numbness, and weakness, especially in extremities

Psoriasis - TNF too high can be brought down with larch tree extract. Skin disorder.

Psoriatic arthritis - Pain, swelling, or stiffness in one or more joints

Pyoderma gangrenosum - deep ulcers that usually occur on the legs

Pure red cell aplasia - bone marrow ceases to produce red blood cells

Rasmussen's encephalitis - rare inflammatory neurological disease with seizures

Raynaud phenomenon - disorder causing reddish discoloration of the fingers, toes

Relapsing polychondritis - inflammation and deterioration of cartilage

Reiter's syndrome - response to an infection in another part of the body

Restless leg syndrome is caused by a cross section of nutrient deficiency

Retroperitoneal fibrosis - proliferation of fibrous tissue in your body

Rheumatoid arthritis - most common, principally attacks flexible synovial joints

Rheumatic fever - illness develops three weeks after a streptococcal infection

Sarcoidosis - inflammatory cells that can form as nodules in multiple organs

Schizophrenia - breakdown of thought processes, deficit of typical emotional responses

Schmidt syndrome - most common form of the polyglandular failure syndromes

Schnitzler syndrome - chronic hives and periodic fever, bone pain and joint pain

Scleritis - affects the white outer coating of the eye

Scleroderma - fibrosis or hardening, vascular alterations, and autoantibodies

Serum Sickness - immune system can mistake the proteins present for harmful antigens

Sjögren's syndrome - destroy the exocrine glands that produce tears and saliva

Spondyloarthropathy - joint disease of the vertebral column

Still's disease - Juvenile rheumatoid arthritis from squalene in vaccinations

Stiff person syndrome - neurologic disorder, progressive rigidity and stiffness

Subacute endocarditis - streptococci bacteria that normally live in the mouth and throat

Susac's syndrome - branch retinal artery occlusions and hearing loss

Sweet's syndrome - skin disease characterized by the sudden onset of fever

Sydenham chorea - see Pandas

Sympathetic ophthalmia - ocular antigens following trauma

Systemic lupus erythematosis - see Lupus erythematosis III, connective tissue disease

Takayasu's arteritis - affects the aorta the main blood vessel leaving the heart

Temporal arteritis - involving large and medium arteries of the head

Thrombocytopenia - decrease of platelets in blood

Tolosa-Hunt syndrome - weakness and paralysis of certain eye muscles

Transverse myelitis - inflammatory process of the spinal cord

Ulcerative colitis - one of two types of idiopathic inflammatory bowel disease "IBD"

Undifferentiated connective tissue disease - Mixed connective tissue disease

Urticarial vasculitis - skin condition characterized by fixed nettle rash lesions that appear histologically as a vasculitis

Vasculitis - disorders that destroy blood vessels by inflammation

Vitiligo -

Wegener's granulomatosis - inflammation of blood vessels that affects small and medium sized vessels in many organs.

All the cures for the above are at your local drugstore. Fibromyalgia is a common autoimmune disease and is one of the most painful to endure. Guaifenesin protocol reduces phosphate in the muscles to reduce pain.

The doctor found the cure for autoimmune by accident while treating a patient in a regular family practice. Because his practice was out in the country, he had more free time for his mind to wander. I think that doctors are engineered to be busy. They go through school their entire lives congratulated for achieving, and then into university, where they are busy studying and working through shifts at the hospital sometimes 40 hours straight saddled with assignments that can be overwhelming. They are occupied by attractive singles looking for a good catch then graduate into debt with a waiting room of patients lined up out the door. Perhaps 3 kids and a spouse who likes to travel, socialize, with a couple of cars, brochures for boats and vacations on the table. The pharmaceutical companies are there to enhance their paychecks. If they happen to drift outside the practice of their manual they are reprimanded and occasionally suspended from practicing medicine. No wonder there haven't been any cures found for disease and the cures that have been found are either ignored or become recipients of scrutiny, ridicule, professional audit, or worse have their place of business raided, equipment and supplies confiscated with guns pointed at their heads as was the case with Dr. Rife, Dr. Hulda Clark in the US and Dr. Eldon Dahl in Canada and enough of these examples to fill several books.

I found FDA to be less than honorable reviewing countless cures for disease available with peer review studies ignored professionally. I've worked with doctors that had their licenses removed and put on QuackWatch. com or they volunteered themselves into retirement practicing outside the official manual. Dr. Ernie Murakami was forced to retire after treating Lyme disease patients with success and saving lives of many, by the College of Physicians and Surgeons of B.C. investigation into his views and practices with regard to the disease. Each province has a similar criminal cabal that serves to protect drug patents and agendas. Doctors who are allowed to practice medicine can only work from a manual so that makes them technicians. Most of the content of "the manual" is misleading which is worse than wrong because it is cloaked in half truths. Just look at the hospitals and the walking dead on the streets, as proof. But society is getting used to dying at age 75 when in cultures that have maintained nourishment in their food absent of toxins, are just learning to play tennis at that age. Results speak louder than words.

Autoimmune is one of the biggest rackets going. The cure is at your local Drug store. I felt the dozen Rheumatologists that I worked with were dangerous because, their objective is to remove your immune system. Their idea of treatment is like unscrewing the light bulb that warns you that your engine oil is low. It is best to go to the cause of the oil light being lit and to add a few quarts/liters of oil instead of unscrewing the warning light and ignoring the problem. Elmore Fudd with a shot gun is the vision I have of a doctor with a prescription pad. Every prescription you take might have 10 consequences. Just watch a commercial on television for an autoimmune drug that goes on to describe the side effects, "if you stop breathing, have chest pains, your eyes start popping out of your head, or you have dizziness, black outs, dry mouth, itchy skin, diarrhea, vomiting, parts of your anatomy falling off, or may cause death", doesn't sound like a road map to recovery and you are expected to pay for this?? Not only with your after tax dollars but with your time.

More about autoimmune

Cement, drywall, wood, or anything that used to be alive is fair food for mold. Mold cannot reliably be tested by doing air samples. Dr. Lin (Microbiologist) from New York confirms a contaminated residence or workplace by putting samples collected from your home and work. A history of dormant and active cycles of mold extracted from your carpets and dust from behind the fridge can be put into petri dishes. These are the places that hide the history of what you have been breathing. He came out with the ERMI standard "Environmental Rating Mold Index" that found that 35% of homes in North America are "sick homes" on a sliding scale of severity from 1-4, 2.5 or less being Ok. Dr Lin's index, found that 35% of all homes in North America will cause Auto-Immune disease and make you sick and for 24% of the population it will be permanent. Auto-Immune disease can easily be confirmed by a blood test. I think Mononucleosis is just a form of Biotoxin Illness or autoimmune, just not listed.

If you use 35% of homes for 24% of the population that are susceptible, that is 1/3 of 24 or 8% of the population with chronic auto-immune and 100% of 35% of the population with temporary auto-immune. That is 40% of people who have at least mild symptoms, half will be significant and only about 10% of the population are diagnosed. Excluding Mexico, there are about 35 million people debilitated and almost 100 million affected as a consequence. North Americans move an average of once every 7 years. My rough calculation is easy to conclude that 40% of the North American population is suffering from some type of autoimmune to some degree of severity. Most of the sufferers are chasing different healing modalities and are attracted to reading this type of book and it is only the most severe that seek a specialist's help. Not one of those patients has a hope with a specialist, because their solution involves partially removing the patient's immune system to relieve pain which leads to further complications of disease and permanent scarring of tissue in affected areas over time. It is also a major cause of lymphoma. I think statistics would be very helpful published in the media about autoimmune and who is reporting the disease and where. This simple exercise gets people thinking and evaluating patterns which will achieve an adoption of treatment for all. I found that most people who have crohn's, or rheumatoid arthritis, or celiac, or lupus, or fibromyalgia, or chronic fatigue, don't know they have autoimmune disease.

Did you ever notice that the same kids at school perhaps 1/2 a dozen were sick a lot, especially in fall and winter? The poisonous gas given off by mold is intended to kill other mold competing for space but can raise auto-immune symptoms of dizziness, muscle aches, lethargy, stomach aches, migraines in 20 minutes confirmed with C3a and C4a blood tests. Patients are at their best at the end of summer and at their worst at the end of winter before the healing rays return. For the northern hemisphere, April 1 is when the effective UVB healing rays return if you are located about 45'N of the equator or reverse for south of the equator. I bet the reason for statistics of autoimmune are low close to equator because homes are absent of vapor barriers and the sun is healing. That's why people with autoimmune or arthritis in their hands, knees and feet seek relief in warm dry places like Arizona and New Mexico.

Incidentally, Autoimmune is the same disease as Chronic Lyme disease and ties into MS. One of the ways to combat Auto-Immune is to sleep with your window cracked open and pull up an extra blanket, get midday sun without suntan lotion because it impedes the benefits of the healing effects of the sun and vitamin D synthesis in the skin. It is the early am and late afternoon sun UVA spectrum sun rays that ages your skin. UVB sun helps to detox and heal your body, so is use of an infrared sauna and infrared heat from fire. When you lower inflammation it increases energy.

Seattle sitting just below 49' N lattitude, has healing midday UVB sun only from April 15 to Sept 1 that peaks at 1pm, 3 weeks off the fall and spring equinox. Sun intensity increases or decreases by 1.8'/week as you go south or north of the equator. Chicago and Toronto start to get beneficial midday sun starting about April 1 to Sept 15. Latitudes between 23'N and 23'S get healing UVB rays year round. You must avoid sun burning to achieve healing effects.

The new term for the disease going into the next century will shift to Biotoxin Illness once the FDA is told to either take a hike or become ethical. They have the statistics and knowledge of the cure for autoimmune monitoring meticulous patient case studies, but they chose to ignore 100% success to an unsuspecting public. Preponderance of evidence is staggering.

NOW is the time to question authority. Profits run this industry and not the welfare of patient care on every level. Information in this book will make prescriptions a thing of the past, "If you weren't born with it you don't need to die with it." Disease and obesity are an option and so is our system where corruption exists on so many levels. There is so much known about Auto-Immune by so few people, it's sad.

In my opinion, the cause and cure for autoimmune using a patient's DNA and a blood lab without question is absolute and the most extraordinary discovery of the century. This is not a free market capitalist society we are living in but perhaps a dictatorship without choice. I prefer freedom of choice, how about you?

Below is an example of how twisted treatment for autoimmune disease is. This is typical of the treatment I was given, that hurt me. Look at this nonsense below and the drug companies are excited to promote this solution for psoriasis. The superior alternative is just 15$ for a couple of months of relief from psoriasis using a vitamin within days. Larch arabinogalactan has been shown to decrease NF-kappaB. Lowering TNF-bl works by "cleaning up" the lymphatic system. I used Larch tree extract supplements

1 or 2 per day from Wellness CA to reduce cause of pain, a symptom of autoimmune.

"Biologics for Psoriasis Article:
Biologics are revolutionizing how psoriasis is treated. Anti-psoriasis biologics have been developed based on current understanding of the abnormal immune system responses that contribute to the disease. As such, they are designed to 'target' specific parts of the immune system. The goal is to weaken or immobilize those features of the immune system that are triggering psoriasis without the adverse side effects that can come from broadly weakening the immune system".

Currently six biologics are U.S. Food and Drug Administration (FDA) approved for approved for psoriasis and/or psoriatic arthritis treatment (generic names are in parentheses):

Amevive (alefacept),
Enbrel (etanercept),
Humira (adalimumab),
Remicade (infliximab),
Simponi (golimumab),

Stelara (ustekinumab)Efalizumab" was withdrawn from the market by its manufacturer in the summer of 2009 because the drug worked too well at taking out your immune system. It was linked to the occurrence of a fatal viral infection of the nervous system called progressive multifocal leukoencephalopathy or PML. Although they differ in the details of their makeup, Enbrel, Remicade, Humira, and Simponi all target the same piece of the immune system - a molecule called Tumor Necrosis Factor-alpha (TNF-alpha). Hence, these drugs are sometimes referred to as 'TNF-inhibitors.' TNF-alpha is an inflammation-promoting substance that is produced abnormally in psoriasis patients.

Amevive targets T-cells, immune cells that accumulate in the skin and joints of psoriasis patients. T-cells are directly and indirectly responsible for the production of a variety of inflammation-causing substances, including TNF-alpha.

Stelara targets interleukin-12 (IL-12) and interleukin-23 (IL-23), immune system molecules found in large amounts at the sites of active psoriasis.

Amevive, Enbrel, Remicade, Humira and Stelara are FDA approved for adults with moderate to severe plaque psoriasis; Enbrel, Remicade, Humira, and Simponi are approved for psoriatic arthritis. Biologics carry strong warnings to alert healthcare professionals of an increased risk of lymphoma and other malignancies in children and adolescents treated with TNF blockers.

End of article. This is nonsense, and I am critical because they know this is nonsense.

The Sequence to Autoimmune or Biotoxin Illness

Biotoxins can cause harm to every facet of our biochemical framework from our immune system to our nervous system and our mitochondria. While all of us are at risk for developing symptoms related to exposure to these biotoxins, 24% individuals are at a greater risk of developing symptoms due to their genetic predisposition. Once exposed, these individuals begin to exhibit symptoms of profound fatigue, joint and muscle pain, memory loss, intolerance to exercise, weight gain, headaches, depression, chronic fatigue, poor word assimilation, loss of sex drive, migraines, and a feeling of emptiness. Some have gastrointestinal dysfunction including diarrhea, bloating, irregular movements and abdominal pain during spikes in mold exposure. HLA-dr (Human Leukocyte Antigen) blood lab is the blueprint to determine the roadmap to recovery.

Biotoxin illness has devastating effects that occur to our immune systems, nervous systems, hormonal systems, mitochondrial systems and detoxification systems as it runs its course. It is a neurological disease that manifests itself physically from exposure to mold. Here is a summary of how biotoxins cause problems to our biological systems.

Stage A: Biotoxin Effects: It starts with exposure to mold. In most people, the biotoxin or neurotoxin is "tagged" and identified by the body's innate immune system and is and removed from the blood by the liver. However, some individuals do not have the genetics measured by the (HLA-dr blood test) gene on chromosome 6, so the neurotoxins are recirculated and remain in the body indefinitely, free to circulate even after removed from exposure. Once in the body, the biotoxins set off a complex cascade of biochemical events. The biotoxin binds to surface receptors (toll receptor) in fat cells. This in turn causes both a continuous and intensification of innate immune system response of cytokines. I have to be conscious of when I am in mold and remove myself. Cytokine response begins within 20 minutes of exposure. Pain and headaches and loss of concentration are the first symptoms and are noticeable.

Stage B: Cytokine Effects: The activated fat cells start to produce leptin, which leads to weight gain that is unresponsive to diet or exercise, while the fat cells are pumping out cytokines, the overload starts to block and damage the leptin receptors in the hypothalamus. Elevated cytokines produce many different symptoms including, headache, muscle ache, unstable temperature and difficulty concentrating. High levels of cytokines result in increased levels of immune related markers such as TNF-b1, MMP-9, IL-1B, and PAI-1. MMP-9 delivers inflammatory elements from the blood into sensitive tissues and can combine with PAI-1 to increase clot formation and arterial blockage. To eliminate cytokine response, I took 2 grams of cholestyramine (Olestyr Rx) 4x/day on an empty stomach. Pain relief started within 30 minutes and I think 15 days or 1 box was enough for me where I didn't see any more improvement but the doctor recommends 30 days.

Stage C: Reduce TRANSFORMING GROWTH FACTOR or TGF-b1, taking 1 tablet of Cozaar at bedtime had a huge impact on lowering pain, so much so, I could stand up out of my wheelchair within a week of taking it. The CSM or Olestyr helped greatly but the Cozaar was amazing. Cozaar is meant to lower high blood pressure and I had low blood pressure, so I took it at bedtime. I only needed 10 days on this med, and it takes about 30 days to kick in for its intended use of lowering blood pressure and is really hard on the kidneys creating pain the next day after taking the first pill. The pain can be taken out in a day with parsley tea. Drink a mug or 2 a day and pain/inflammation relief works fast. It's good for Dialysis patients.

Stage D: Reduced VEGF: Vascular endothelial growth factor is responsible for helping regulate blood vessel integrity. The elevated cytokine levels in the capillaries attract white blood cells, leading to restricted blood flow and lowered oxygen levels in the tissues because of inflammation. Reduced VEGF leads to fatigue, muscle cramps and shortness of breath. This marker was not a problem for me.

Stage E: Immune System Effects: Patients with the "24%" immune related genes usually develop inappropriate immune responses which may include antibodies to myelin basic protein from fungal infections, gliadin wheat-like allergies and cardiolipins that affect blood clotting. I found that with autoimmune or biotoxin illness, evidence of my immune system crash was just a break in the skin, where I would get boils and became easily susceptible to colds and occasionally pneumonia.

Stage F: MSH: Melanocyte stimulating hormone blood test is important because it is a master controller of immune response. It is the most potent anti-inflammatory compound in your body that comes from the hypothalamus. The hypothalamus is involved in several functions of the body including:

Autonomic Function Control
Endocrine Function Control
Homeostasis
Motor Function Control
Food and Water Intake Regulation
Sleep-Wake Cycle Regulation

Reduced alpha-melanocyte stimulating hormone (MSH) production results in poor quality sleep. Endorphin production is suppressed which leads to chronic pain and intolerance to pain. Lack of MSH can cause malabsorption or "leaky gut," which further weakens and deregulates the immune system. White blood cells begin to lose regulation of cytokine response, and infections easily occur. Recovery from infections and of exercised muscles grinds to a halt. I responded well to VIP to raise MSH, but not enough. Leptin is the fat cell hormone that binds to MSH contributing to weight gain.

Stage G: about Antibiotic Resistant Staph Bacteria: Reduced MSH also allows resistant staph Marcons to flourish deep inside the nose. The bacteria live on the surface of the tissue, deep inside the nose and are the major clue you are living in mold. These bacteria further compound the problem by producing exotoxins A and B that cleave MSH, that further decrease MSH levels. At this point, the downward spiral starts. MSH is a key hormone you need to be healthy. Rofact or Rifampin (in the US) is a bactericidal antibiotic drug, as a cream on a Q-tip pushed far up your nose into each nostril helps control the staph Marcons and associated headaches. VIP or Vaso Intestinal Peptide was magic and is pricey.

Stage H: Pituitary Hormone Effects: Reduced MSH decreases pituitary production of antidiuretic hormone ADH which leads to thirst, frequent urination, neurally-mediated hypotension NMH, low blood volume, and electric shocks from static electricity. I would get huge jolts of shocks from my wheelchair. While sex hormone production falls off, the pituitary may increase the production of cortisol and ACTH in the early stages of illness, then drop to abnormally low, or low normal ranges.

Cortisol testing is done by salivary testing throughout the day, and is a stress hormone released by adrenal gland. DHEA is another stress hormone that complements cortisol. My treatment with autoimmune and DHEA/testosterone helped with my recovery. Testosterone varies based upon blood testing and to androgenic hormone that seems to change inversely to cortisol.

CRP: blood test is a non-specific marker of inflammation on a general level throughout the body.

ESR: blood test another non-specific marker of inflammation.

TNF Tumor Necrosis Factor: an inflammatory cytokine that gets turned on by biotoxins.

MMP-9(Matrix Metalloproteinase): another inflammatory cytokine.

PAI-1: Plasminogen activator inhibitor.

Anticardiolipins: When elevated there will be an issue with blood clotting.

Toxic Mold poisoning is the single most deadly element in the Health Matrix there is for sickness, disease and death of anything else combined in health. Smoking is nowhere near what toxic mold does to humans. In Manitoba, Canada I hear there is a community, that has a high incidence of Lou Gherig's disease, and this is most probably due to fresh water algae, that when blooms causes headaches, sleeplessness, body aches and deterioration in health of this disease.

Biotoxin Summary

The "Biotoxin Pathway" illustrates an ongoing, increasing cascade of events that starts with exposure to biotoxins or mold in those individuals who are genetically susceptible. The biotoxin then binds to toll receptors in fat-cells and also cells that line blood vessels, resulting in the production of proteins called cytokines which are involved in immune response of inflammatory symptoms. Cytokines recognize invaders and recruit additional cytokines in response.

It is the biotoxin itself called neurotoxins that continuously signals the body to produce more cytokines. It is this cytokine production that makes us feel unwell. Excess cytokines result in flu-like symptoms, body aches, temperature fluctuations, cognitive difficulties and other symptoms. It made me feel like I got hit by a bus. This increase in cytokines has further negative effects.

VEGF (vascular endothelial growth factor) is often reduced which leads to fatigue and reduced blood flow. Hypoperfusion results in a reduction in blood flow, which then starves the cells for nutrients and oxygen. There is also an increase in MMP9 (matrix metalloproteinase) as the cytokine causes the white blood cells to release MMP9. MMP9 is a great marker for the presence of excess cytokines.

MMP9 is responsible for removing inflammatory compounds out of the blood and into the brain which causes plaque formations similar to those seen in MS patients. In Lyme disease, MMP9 levels sometimes skyrocket as the result of treatment with antibiotics and the resulting bacterial die-off in what is referred to as a Herxheimer reaction. If you give a Lyme-infected person antibiotics or better oxygen treatment and they are not HLA-susceptible, they generally have a regular recovery.

There are three key types of antibodies observed in those with biotoxin-associated illnesses. These are myelin (the protective sheath around nerve cells) antibodies, gliadin (a protein found in gluten) antibodies, and cardiolipin antibodies which impact circulation in the small blood vessels.

With Lyme disease there are increases determined by blood tests which reflect activation of the complement system in C3a and C4a. C4a levels become elevated as early as twelve hours after a tick bite. In the case of those with a mold-susceptible HLA type, C4a significantly increases within four hours after re-exposure to a moldy environment, my experience is 30 minutes. C4a can be a helpful blood test in determining whether a remediated home is still a danger for someone with biotoxin susceptibility. If C4a levels have been reduced via remedies and C4a levels rise upon reintroduction, it is a sign that the environment is not safe for the patient.

Leptin is a hormone made by fat cells which helps to regulate the storage of fat. When leptin increases as the result of a biotoxin exposure and MSH (alpha melanocyte stimulating hormone) is reduced, people become obese and weight loss is next to impossible. Weight gain is related to exposure to Lyme disease, or to mold/ biotoxins.

MSH, made in the hypothalamus, is the most potent anti-inflammatory there is. It is responsible for regulating innate immune response and is involved in many hormone pathways. MSH is at the heart of the "Biotoxin Pathway". Many negative effects result when MSH is low. The FDA won't release this essential hormone to the public. MSH is low in about 97% of autoimmune and Lyme patients.

When MSH levels are low, people have problems falling sleep, have chronic pain, they experience leaky gut syndrome, their recovery from illness is delayed, they develop multiple antibiotic resistant coagulase negative staph colonization (MARCoNS), they have frequent thirst as a result of lowered anti-diuretic hormone (ADH), they have a loss of libido due to a lowering of sex hormones and there are more.

MSH is involved in the production of melatonin and endorphins. This resulting lack of endorphins increases sensitivity to pain. MSH regulates the protective cytokine responses in the blood, skin, digestive tract, and respiratory membranes. Lowered MSH results in abnormalities in production of cortisol and fluctuations in ACTH (adrenocorticotropic hormone) which regulates adrenal function. It is when the biotoxin or autoimmune illness disrupts the production of MSH that so many of the symptoms emerge. When looking at the results of lab tests for reduced MSH and increased C4a, using these markers, the diagnostic accuracy is compelling.

With "Biotoxin Pathway" understood, recovery is clear. Cholestyramine (CSM) is a resin that has a positive charge that binds to negatively charged neurotoxins for excretion through the digestive tract. Without CSM, these toxins are reabsorbed and continue to re-circulate indefinitely. Though gastrointestinal side effects are not uncommon and include constipation and other digestive issues, only 10% of patients stop using CSM. It is usually a symptom of poor gut flora. This can be corrected using the IBS tip in chapter 8 and probiotics. If CSM therapy is used while there is ongoing exposure to mold/biotoxins, the patient will remain ill.

If there is an ongoing infection, with Lyme patients, C4a will often fall but slowly rises back to pre-treatment values after an initial of treatment. This may be an indication that spirochete bacteria are still present and will be an indication that further oxygen/rife therapy is justified. A rapid rise of C4a back to pre-treatment levels may also suggest that mold/ biotoxins are still present.

Treatment for biotoxins will often incorporate targeted gene therapy using Actos. Actos is a drug approved for the treatment of diabetes that also has a significant number of benefits for those with biotoxin associated illness. Beyond being anti-inflammatory, Actos lowers leptin, lowers MMP9, raises VEGF, and positively affects other markers.

Actos is an important discovery in treating biotoxin illnesses, in fact, for people with Lyme disease and chronic Lyme, CSM by itself may create a significant intensification of a Herxheimer's reaction. This intensification is observed in over 50% of patients and is the result of a cytokine storm. This storm is effectively blocked by pretreatment of 10 days using Actos. This is a very important part of treating a biotoxin illness in someone with Lyme disease. CSM alone is generally more difficult for that patient to tolerate and less successful in terms of eventual outcome. The benefits of CSM therapy are limited to the binding of toxins, it cannot do more than that.

Unfortunately, Actos doesn't work if the patient continues to consume a high-glycemic index diet. The treatment, uses a no-amylose diet that restricts the intake of carbohydrates, which contain amylose. These consist of wheat, rice, oats, barley, rye, bananas, and any vegetable that grows beneath the ground except for onions and garlic.

If you correct MARCoNS nasal colonization, VEGF deficiencies, and avoid gliadin, treatment with CSM and Actos will result in more than 92% of patients showing a 75% or greater reduction in symptoms within 30 days.

Dr. Zamboni's method opens up blood flow to the body and returns drastic improvement to body mobility for MS patients. We need to change the building codes to eliminate mold in homes and at work. There are many other doctors who can come forward with their cures that can't or who are afraid to because the FDA and their agencies will destroy them. This scenario happened to Dr. Burzynski of Houston Texas with his method of curing cancer, but there have been many more before him. Americans are in survival mode and over half are sick and going bankrupt. It's not about being right or wrong, obedient vs immoral. Doing chemo and ignoring the cure for 170 autoimmune diseases, all cancer and unhealthy weight is like watching society running toward a cliff blindfold not knowing the options available. This book is an effort to pull down the blind fold and offer real choice to change the system to one without an agenda. Truth has no agenda. There are no risks to taking high density nutrient meal replacements, juicing organic vegetables and eliminating toxins. The effort you put forth will get you to thrive with energy and save you a ton of money and time! Forget about ego and promote compassion. This will begin to end suffering for hundreds of millions of people. This is real, this is what I care about.

Mastering Leptin by Byron Richards.

I had a big mix up at the store. When the woman said "strip down facing me," she was referring to my credit card.

How do you put a zebra into a refrigerator?
Answer chapter 4.

Chapter 4

Hormones for life

Hormones rank 2nd as the most important of the 5 elements to achieve super immunity, raise pH, lower inflammation, lower excess weight and to get yourself off medications, avoid disease and health issues associated with old age. Hormones are the "software" of the body. They direct a number of bodily functions. People think it is a drug but it is an essential nutrient that everyone over 40 needs to have in their veins to thrive. Hormones give life, it is what your body needs.

There are really 4 main hormones to focus on, 2 for men and 2 for women. Women have Dhea and testosterone which are 2 others added in trace amounts where blood tests permit, added to the main ingredients of progesterone and estrogen. For persons 35 and younger hormones are usually not an issue but don't rule them out.

Not only do hormones decrease inflammation but slow the aging process and effectively. The older you are the fewer hormones you have and this is why your body declines and aging accelerates. This is when cellular death increases and cellular rejuvenation decreases. It is this ratio that is the principal of aging and it can be manipulated with hormones available circulating in your blood stream. Hormones interrelate to one another. If one is up the other might be down and if one hormone is deficient, this can affect the ratio of other hormones. Amounts of one hormone can affect the protein binding of another. Bioidentical hormone replacement is done with several hormones simultaneously because of hormone interaction.

Your thyroid is one of many hormone glands in your body. Hormones control almost every facet of your body from your thinking, sugar regulation, weight, muscles, digestion, bones, mood, and personality. The power of hormones is significant. Hormones are in control and make big changes to your body, just look at what hormones can do during pregnancy.

I observed several adults over 50 who looked early 40's, 10 years younger, in their step, skin, bounce, hair, sparkly eyes, wit, energy, and frequency or mood, and every measure of youth you could see and hear. The diet of these 50+ individuals was average at best, yet they never got sick, depressed or anything less than bubbly. With the science of bio identical hormones circulating in their blood, collagen, botox and plastic surgery concerns were far out on the horizon for these people if ever. They didn't have the benefit of ever doing an organ cleanse, or a good diet but had the sex drive and energy of a 30 year old, morning, noon, and night. Hormones drop off 1-3% a year over the age of 30. You can maintain a youthful look into your 50's by taking birth control pills but it can be risky as they impact your progesterone production in your ovaries.

Adreanal Glands & Their Essential Bodily Functions

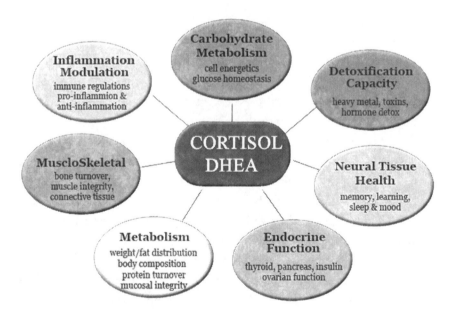

Adrenal Hormones

CORTISOL, is the hormone responsible for immune regulation and energy boosting. People exposed to long term stress and autoimmune can burn out their adrenal glands and be chronically tired as a result.

DHEA helps with libido and may also convert for bone and muscle building. DHEA is an androgen, a precursor to testosterone and falls off a cliff after age 21. About 50mg/tablet/daily is typical for adult males. DHEA must be present to oppose the conversion of testosterone to estrogen if testosterone is unopposed.

PREGNENOLONE is good for memory and not considered important.

ESTROGEN

Must be matched with progesterone to be safely taken. As women age it becomes more and more important.

GROWTH HORMONE is completely gone from your system by the time you are 21 years old. It requires injections. Human Growth Hormone is great at increasing muscle mass and reducing fat.

LEPTIN Lack of sleep also decreases levels of the fat regulating hormone leptin while increasing the hunger hormone ghrelin.

MELATONIN is best known for its sleep inducing properties. It helps with jet lag, and is deactivated by light where you sleep. The pill form is natural and can be dissolved underneath the tongue at bedtime. This hormone also drops off after age 21. It is sold as an OTC over the counter med in 3 and 5 mg tablets. It is a sleep inducer that is natural to the body.

PROGESTERONE is a hormone deficient in most women. Women with underactive thyroids are also progesterone deficient. Estrogen mimickers called xenoestrogens found in plastics, parabens, are suppressing ovarian production of progesterone. It is the most important hormone to women. It is typically taken on the last 15 days of your cycle and daily if you are post menopause. Taking the pill to stop contraception decreases ovarian ability to make progesterone which makes you susceptible to ovarian cancer if taken over a long period of time.

TESTOSTERONE is needed to be manly and its production falls off when men hit 40. A host of old age symptoms begin following the decline. Women need testosterone too in small amounts. For women its benefits are libido, bone strength, muscles, memory, initiative, and self-esteem. The healthiest testosterone is in a cream. The injectable type is made of horse urine and not a healthy version of testosterone. Cortisol is the stress hormone that is the polar opposite to Testosterone. It blocks the Testosterone hormone. The estrogen mimickers from plastics raise obesity levels and lowers Testosterone levels. Eugenics is now called "planned parenthood". Alcohol eats testosterone and statin drugs dissolve it.

THYROID For thyroid function, iodine is the top supplement for health that there is and is deficient world wide. Women require 2-3x more iodine than men because of breast tissue. The RDA or recommended daily allowance is 100x too small and is only enough to prevent goiters. Read the book by Dr Brownstein and Dr Abraham on thyroid research.

VITAMIN D is considered a hormone. It is the second most effective anti inflammatory supplement. Vitamin D begins to work when taken at 5000iu/day when you don't get your minimum ½ hour of sun. Vitamin D deficiency is like that of iodine. Vitamin D should be given to newborns and taken by all children, women and men daily.

HGH is injectable peptide taken weekly and is good for increasing muscle and decreasing fat.

IGF is an injectable anabolic steroid.

MSH is alpha Melanocyte Stimulating Hormone is wonderful for sense of well-being, prevents sunburning, decreases pain sensitivity and gets damaged from symptoms of autoimmune. There is a cosmetic type of MSH that can enhance tanning for those susceptible to sun burning. It is an injectable peptide done weekly.

Note: For males it's dangerous to dispense testosterone on its own, unopposed to DHEA (dehydroepiandrosterone). DHEA is an important endogenous steroid hormone and stops the testosterone from turning to estrogen and becoming a toxic cancer causing agent. Prostate cancer is common among those that take testosterone on its own without DHEA. It can be taken on its own everyday throughout the month but Testosterone is best taken 3 weeks on and one week off so that your body is encouraged to continue making its own testosterone. It is best to go to a bio available Hormone Specialist MD for hormones, for blood tests and prescriptions for both men and women.

If you don't have the 750$ for this important treatment, for females I am aware of Estro 500 estrogen and PC 30 progesterone off the internet from Amazon.com or Amazon.ca in Canada for about 80$ a month or two of supply for females. Estrogen or Estro 500 is the female equivalent to testosterone. Never take it on its own unless prescribed by a bio identical hormone specialist. Regular family practice doctors don't, in my opinion, have the knowledge to reliably dispense prescriptions for hormones. The doctors I met are dispensing testosterone without Dhea! Eeks.

Youthful looking ladies in their late 40's take progesterone on the last 15 days of their cycle and others are taking progesterone daily post menopausal. If you take estrogen it would be best to take it less, perhaps 3 weeks a month because of the estrogen you absorb from BPA and the more toxic BPS used in plastic drinking containers and linings of beer cans and soup cans. Parabens are found in some suntan lotions and underarm deodorants which are all estrogen mimickers acting like estrogen but in a toxic version to the body that cause cancer. Best to buy organic consumer products. Talk to your doctor or find one who is versed.

It was interesting to watch Suzanne Sommers do the television circuit promoting the wonderful health benefits of hormones for her book. She obviously had a youthful glow years ahead of her peers. The spin propaganda machine embraced the obvious fact of the immense benefits of youthful hormones and spun it around to make it look like a waste of money. The pharmaceutical interests recognized a threat from Suzanne's ideas about the benefits of bioidentical hormones that would erode their sales of drugs related to old age like, anti depressants, constipation, pain pills, sleeping pills, heart and cholesterol and hypertension medication. With the adoption of the internet the suppression is getting harder to spin.

Hormones are one of the five elements of health that if in balance help prevent disease by enhancing cellular rejuvenation. This is partially why kids can play all day and eat fast food full of toxins void of nutrients and still get up and play the next day with energy. Children have seed energy similar to a seed in nature, as seen in wheat grass. Wheat grass has nutritional density as a sprout but once it starts to mature that density is lost so wheat grass is harvested young perhaps only 6-9 inches tall. The external source of nutrition is not as important under the age of 35 as it is once your hormones begin to fall off. At about age 30, you start to lose hormones and that is when aging begins to reveal itself. This is the point at which the balance of cellular rejuvenation begins to lose the war against cellular death. After age 35 you begin to lose a pound of muscle a year to fat, assuming the same lifestyle is maintained. After age 40 the aging process begins to accelerate.

A hormone replacement program to set the hormone blood levels to that of a 30 year old is the level achieved where the benefits of cellular repair and rejuvenation initially reverses the appearance of age, by my estimate 5 years and then aging slows down significantly close to half.

- If you are 55 years old with 30 year old hormones, you might look about 45.
- If you are 65 year old with 30 year old hormones, you might look 50-55.

I met patients who regretted going off hormones in their mid-70's under the advice of their doctor. With the suspension of hormone therapy they quickly began to look their age and developed old age symptoms and health issues quickly as a consequence. These patients were warned by their doctor through guidance of unethical science to get off hormones which the patient later regretted.

I suggest everyone have their hormones in balance, Testosterone with DHEA for men and Estrogen with Progesterone for women and bio-available which means that there are free hormones available in the blood stream measured by blood tests for cellular rejuvenation. Once off hormones aging accelerates and the symptoms of irritability, sleeplessness, fatigue and low energy, brain fog, lower vitality, wrinkles, low collagen, aches and pains, and disease begin to emerge. Hormones in balance keep the need for cosmetic surgery, psychiatrists, collagen injections, and botox irrelevant. Hormone replacement is best done following autoimmune disease and cancer. Hormone levels get damaged with inflammation and the cytokine response of the innate immune system.

An employee at a hospital in her 50's experiencing menopause wouldn't consider hormones because she was already on too many drugs chronically as it was. Taking hormones would likely help her eliminate most of her medications if she consulted a bioidentical hormone specialist, and likely put her in a more pleasant mood. It's hard to be pleasant when you are inflamed and on several medications.

Bioidentical hormones are nothing less than amazing to enhance your health and to lower inflammation. It is best done at the end of your recovery and absent of autoimmune sypmtoms and cancer.

Answer:
Open the refrigerator and take out the penguin and put in the zebra and close the door. This tests your ability to think through your previous actions.

Chapter 5

Nutrition - our food and water

The trouble with our health today is that you need Whimis training and a 1-800 Poison-Control phone number ready to shop at a grocery store today and convenience stores are worse. I walk through the aisles of a grocery store and can't find anything that isn't inflammatory and doesn't contribute to obesity and disease aside from your organic produce and in most stores and restaurants, organic is rare. They say that the outside aisles of the grocery store are the aisles where you can find healthy food and drink, but those isles are just "less bad for you". If you look into the ingredients that make up some of those products in the "good aisles", it would turn your stomach. Unless the product is organic, the nutrition has been removed and toxins have been creatively loaded up by high tech engineering.

Organic is just normal food from 60 years ago. If you have arthritis, run long distance, want to thrive, or have disease, you need to do more than eat organic food. Organic lacks the broad spectrum of nutrients and intensity of nutrition to properly use nutrient as a tool to wellness and weight loss. It will help stabilize and help to maintain good health as a base but will not get you to the top of wellness. The superior benefit of organic is that it is absent of toxins. "Less fat and diet" generally means, more fattening, processing, unnatural, and more inflammatory. Low energy is a function of high inflammation and pain, period. The cheapest prices are always found on the products with the highest toxins and the lowest nutritional content.

Nutrients give life and toxins remove life. Health is an equation of these ratios. The best nutrient your body needs is the one you are lowest in, so why not give your body all of them? Nutrition is the 3rd most important element in the Matrix that contributes to raising your blood pH, your immunity and lowering your inflammation. I argue that nutrition is only the 3rd most important element because kids with abundant hormones (2nd most important element), can play soccer and run all day on fast food, candy and fresh air and do it with energy. I compared kids playing and nutrition to like a seed of grass in nature. Both only need water. After you turn 35, as health sustaining hormones fall off is when your food source becomes more important assuming you are out of mold and symptoms of autoimmune. The kids seem to live off the seed of life and adults over 35 rely on their nutrition of what they are putting in their bodies. I found that adults over 50 who had never cleansed and only ate a mediocre diet, thrived, while adults with the same lifestyle without hormones didn't fare very well. With nutrition, understand that nutrition is your Life Force energy to thrive. If you add cleansing of your liver and kidneys as well, to a good diet and hormones, you might as well say goodbye to health care costs, antibiotics, lost time at work, and you might be able to use Obama's 17,000 rules on health to heat your house this winter in your fireplace? Who would have thought that cures to obesity, inflammation, pain, and disease prevention and oxygen, were to be found in aisles of a health food store?

I found that the cure for disease was so easy. For everyone, we used the same protocol and varied slightly to a personal program with one or two supplements. No more than a dozen products were needed for the worst, but for most everyone just 2 items is enough for people to thrive.

With the invention of the computer and access to the internet, those of us who know about healthcare or had to in order to live, have gotten together, especially in the last 5 years to put together a wealth of information that works. Access to these alternative products are well under way to being shut down today along with internet users sharing this information. We want to share with people this underground health care system and protect the doctors who can deliver oxygen therapy for cancer, the cure for autoimmune, and remarkable breakthroughs for other diseases.

Topics to be your own nutritionist:

Life Force Energy - Is the absolute amount of energy of the food you are eating. Toxins reduce efficiency of nutrient absorption, interfere with cellular integration of nutrients into the cells and with organ function's ability to process nutrients.

Nutrient Density - Expressed % as a value of Life Sustaining Nutrients vs Waste. Nutrient density = Nutrients/ Calories. 114 nutrients divided by 250 calories is intense and diverse nutrition. Meal replacement has the equivalent nutrition estimated to be 10 meals in a 12 oz. glass of water. Juicing has similar characteristics of nutrient concentration to accelerate health to a point of thriving, way beyond worries of disease. Juicing has the added benefit of detoxing your body. Beets work well for the liver and parsley for the kidneys.

Bioavailability - Is the body's ability to absorb nutrients in their composition into your cells. Probiotics and digestive enzymes assist with absorption. It is your body's ability to recognize the nutrients of what you are eating. Iodine matched with iodide has an 800% advantage of bioavailability over iodine matched with potassium which is the type commonly sold in health food stores. Iodine protects you from radiation exposure and should be taken daily by everyone. Employees who work at nuclear power plants should take note. Iodine limits radiation uptake into the thyroid and no exposure to radiation is best.

Fractality - the scientific measure of life and death of food and of people expressed as both octives (death) and fractals (life or Qi).

Organic vs non organic - Knowing where to shop for organic. It is a chore at first but will be rewarding.

Grocery store vs Health food store - Importance of not just the food you eat but the products that are used against your skin that are contributing to inflammation and obesity can't be ignored.

Municipal water - Understand how toxic municipal McWater is. Avoid drinking chemically toxic water, and showering in it is worse for those of you want to get healthy and stay healthy.

A handmade formula I consumed which is batched in small volumes, has the highest Life Force energy available on the planet, and if they served it daily in a hospital recovery would be nothing less than spectacular. If people ate this food throughout communities there would be a thin line of people needing the use of a hospital. The profile of patients would be the expectant mothers, the trauma patients and the aged.

People are in hospitals because of poor health or trauma. The patients suffering with trauma and requiring surgery would recover 2x faster on this high density nutrient diet and that is a conservative estimate. I saw patients bumbling around with the same health issues for 6 months that could have been resolved in 2 weeks with cleansing meal replacement. I proved it to the shock and awe of the surgeons, who took the name of the product with note pad and pen at my bedside. The other patients in the hospital are there because their life force energy is so low they can't live without assisted living or medical intervention, that can dramatically be improved within a couple of weeks. Their immune systems have been compromised from poor diet and toxins from medications, food, and water intake accumulated over time. Their muscles are so inflamed like rust, they can't walk without an aid. For some their health flirts with the seasons of summer with symptoms of autoimmune. Winter drains life force energy and summer replenishes it. Autoimmune patients are best at the end of summer and are at their worst at the end of winter.

Poor health accumulates over a factor of time. Over time there is a gentle break down of cellular health as a result of inflammation that is present from a deficiency of nutrition, I call an imbalance. Weak genes and poor health choices exacerbate the toxic accumulations of poor diet. Poor diet exists in every product in a grocery store and is almost impossible to avoid for most.

Is your food LIFE SUSTAINING or is it POISON?

The concept is simple, if what you are consuming is not "life sustaining", then it is toxic and leads to dysfunction of your cells in your body, your organs, your energy, your mood, your weight, and your mind. Toxins give you a negative Life Force that your body must then exert energy to rid of unable to integrate into cells, and elimination success is not 100%, so it is accumulated. All food, drink, people and even trees have Life Force energy. A patient with 0% Life Force is someone who is dead. A patient with 10% life force might be someone in hospital with severe pneumonia. 20% life force might be someone who has been just discharged from hospital. Most people live in a range of 30-60% and the vibrant people, I suggest, are those thriving at 60-80% of their potential. Very few are above in my estimate, perhaps the pro athletes and performers? Patients who have kidney failure or have liver disease will have their Life Force energy pulled down by that organ. Misery loves company and an acute illness brings down the entire body's energy.

I propose, that eating food that is exceptionally life sustaining, void of toxins, would be a great choice for those that want to get on the elevator of health going up. The sky is the limit. I haven't come across anyone, even vegetarians who are eating organic, drinking healthy water and exercising regularly, who didn't benefit from consuming a protein meal replacement who had found their limit with their current protocols, where their energy and vibrancy improved significantly. If you want to see healthy people, stand outside an organic grocery store. The unhealthiest people I've seen are walking the regular discount supermarket aisles looking for the cheapest prices. The cheapest prices are always found on the products with the highest toxins and the lowest nutrient content. Why is that?

Food that has the highest life force is food that is alive. Buddhist monks try to eat food that is alive and that is the concept of success behind being a vegetarian because this is a low inflammatory diet. Buddhist monks can touch their toes at age 80 and to achieve that, they must have low inflammation throughout their bodies. Avoid meat that isn't organic and try to avoid meat from a 4 legged animal, it is inflammatory and makes your body acidic.

My Meal Replacement

I didn't need to concern myself with nutrition for recovery because I relied on high density protein meal replacement, which is like a health food store in a pail. In one glass of water, I could put in 4 serving scoops and receive the equivalent of 10 meals of nutrition. It has more than enough readily available daily protein in 2 servings am/pm for the day and 77 minerals, along with digestive enzymes, probiotics, fermented live cell grown multi ascorbate vitamin C, 11x more actively bioavailable than what you can buy in a store. The phytosterols which are plant fats known as sterols and steroline have been shown to boost the immune system so well that they stop the decline of T-cells in AIDS patients. They also help to fight cancer, tuberculosis, psoriasis, allergies, lupus, and symptoms of autoimmune. The meal replacement helps protect against oxidized cholesterol, and the side effects of chemo and radiation. Phytosterols help modulate the functions of lymphocytes called T-cells which fight tumors helping to inhibit cancer cell division, viruses and bacteria. Phytosterols reduce cholesterol, help protect bone marrow, and are helpful against auto immune disease. The formula contains all forms of vitamin B and E, iodine, fiber, carotenoids, metal chelators, polysaccharides, phospholipids, poly-phenols, and tocotrienols. The formula contained 120 naturally occurring antioxidants, as a rice based protein. Note: about 70% of all food grown on our planet is rice. It is estimated that more than 60 million tons of rice bran are thrown out each year due to being rancid which begins to set in 12 hours after the bran is milled from the rice. The bran contains more than 70% of the nutrient value of whole rice. It appears to be the most diversified and dense nutrient in the food chain.

Positive changes with the formula I consumed in a glass of water are better blood glucose levels, increased energy, improved circulation in the extremities, and a decrease in numbness due to neuropathy. An improvement in vision and lowering of blood pressure was noticed while on this formula. It is known to reduce insulin requirements of 20-40% and you can double that if you were to flush and clean your liver. This formula has also been proven to lower PSA levels, help with herniated disks, swollen prostate, skin conditions, erectile dysfunction, reduced bruising, and gives you healthier skin and hair within a month. Its presence improves the condition of every cell in your body it comes in contact with.

As well as the protein meal replacement I ate organic fruits and vegetables. I chose to add iodine, chlorella, 10,000 ui of vitamin D, EFA's, high quality tumeric, and everyone should daily. I did add Isashake from Isagenix.com, Vega Protein, and Progressive meal replacements on the counter for occasional use. By juicing organic vegetables and apples, I brought my level of health up to another level that was unbelievable to anyone who hasn't tried it. I also cleansed my kidneys and liver (chapter 6).

We can change emotions immediately to deal with stress - we can change our DNA in 2 weeks on this diet.

Quick List to start:

Drink non-toxic water distilled which is 100% fluoride free or reverse osmosis which is 90% free. Most bottled water now contains chlorine and/or fluoride and is toxic in any amount and is more toxic than drinking water out of tap this way because of the plastic contamination of some 44 chemicals found in trace amounts.

Eat non-toxic food that is organic. "Fresh food" is very often toxic and absent of nutrition.

Eat high density nutrient meal replacement every day for proteins and amino acids to satisfy critical nutritional requirements. It is a health food store in a pail containing all the vitamins and minerals.

Eat and buy only organic products, including toothpaste, sunscreen, salt, ketchup, laundry detergent, soaps, lotions and underarm deodorant that touch your skin.

Juice vegetables and make fruit smoothies or eat them raw along with salads. You can't get enough organic vegetables!

Consume a few supplements, EFA's known as fatty acids (Omega and Krill oils suppress fat food cravings). Iodine is mandatory daily and prevents 20 different diseases and ailments. Himalayan sea salt, Vitamin D 5-10,000iu/day, tumeric, chlorella or spirulina, coconut oil for cooking daily only from a health food store to ensure quality can replace margarine and butter.

Maximize nutrient absorption into your blood and cells with probiotics and digestive enzymes.

Avoid food within ½ hour of drinking coffee, soda, alcohol, smoking, and never use a microwave!

Avoid Aspartame, it is toxic and is the feces of Ecoli.

Avoid fat free food because it is fattening.

Avoid GMO like the plague, it puts your internal organs into inflammation and begins to shut down their function, for some, quicker than others. Watch for symptoms of pain in your lower right gut and in your kidneys as a sign of Genetically Modified food poisoning. GMO is even in baby formula now! (see chap 8)

Avoid any vaccination like the plague. It causes autism in all that take it, to a varying degree of intensity. It also causes autoimmune disease symptoms and for some permanent, and it has been proven to weaken immune systems of all who take it and make people sick more often by an average of 400% on one study of 19,000 children. (see chapter 8)

Cleanse your liver every season of the year and kidneys monthly with parsley tea. (see cleanses chap 6).

Consider bioidentical hormones after age 40 to slow your aging, these are not drugs but are essential like a nutrient.

Cardio exercise in the morning, and daily to stay in shape for 12-20 minutes followed by a protein drink. Exercise should be left for the last 20 lbs of your weight loss recovery.

Pay attention to the importance of sleep. Avoid basements and try melatonin (otc) under your tongue before bedtime.

Consider aloe vera gel, apple cider vinegar, cinnamon, ginger, electrolytes. Nano-colloidal silver occasionally under the tongue and swallowed for additional benefits is a great chelator and boost immunity.

Take stabilized oxygen daily. There are 2 types first, h2o2 food grade that kills disease that should only be taken temporarily and there is a stabilized oxygen with 11% ozone you should take daily that kills diseased cells gently and can be taken with food. To replace coffee put 11% stabilized oxygen in your glass of organic juiced vegetables. This will boost your IQ, vision and energy before a run or an exam within 30 minutes. It is a dietary supplement sold at your health food store. Oxygen is a natural and non-toxic bacteriocide, virucide and fungicide. Oxygen also helps the body metabolize nutrients.

All this reduces inflammation if you are out of mold and absent of autoimmune symptoms. 6 drops of h2o2 in a gallon of milk should keep it fresh in the refrigerator for 6 months.

Note: It has been discovered through testing that, a disturbing number of supplements have no bioavailability to your body, and are nothing more than ground up rocks marketed as healthy, sold in non-health food stores.

Life Force

If you are sick and want to get better, or if you are healthy and want to get healthier, food and water with high Life Force need to be consumed when possible. It is like an equation. Energy in, energy out, or garbage in, garbage health out. There is fast food that has negative Life Force, and by consuming it, will take energy out of your body trying to excrete it. Water that is delivered to your tap using fluoride or chlorine has negative Life Force. Municipal water delivered to your tap using h2o2 (oxygen food grade) has a positive Life Force energy and is healthy to drink. You should use h2o2 for your wells instead of the poison "chlorine".

Your body is very patient and tries very hard to process, use, and place the nutrients you give it. Food can suck energy out of you, if you are eating this type of low vibrational food called, angry DNA. This type of food is called food replacement and is typical of fast food restaurants and convenience stores. The next better is called food substitute, where nutrients have been drastically reduced by processing, and that food is found in abundance in grocery stores like milk that has been pasteurized. The third type is regular food and the forth is super food like chlorella and spirulina. Organic is the definition of real regular food. Organic food is real food because the life cycle in the growth of it hasn't been broken by pesticides, hormones, radiation, pasteurization, processing or adulteration.

Food - Bioavailability of Nutrients vs Waste

To be healthy you need to eat food that is bio available to your cells, which means your body recognizes it as quality food, with little waste and is high in Life force. They are really quite similar in meaning both referencing nutrition in optimal format, but in our society it's easier said than done. There is a sad lack of restaurants and grocery stores serving organic fare. If you are one of these entrepreneurs and you want to increase business, try serving organic to the new wave of customers coming. This is a push/pull marketing concept. Instead of pushing your same old, same old menu that everyone else on the strip is serving, try putting together an organic menu to serve the new wave of customers that don't want to waste their time chewing on food that leaves them with little health benefit and an irritated gut. I ask the readers to get out there and ask the restaurants and grocery store managers to start stocking more organics once the truth gets out about the science behind organic is properly reported.

You get all the protein and amino acids you need in a day from meal replacements but come up short in vegetables, salads and fruits. Juicing organic fruits and vegetables is an ideal way to go! The juice from a juicer separates the raw nutrients out of carrots, apples, lemons, celery, kale, cucumbers, and beets into a glass and by drinking it this way. It absorbs into your blood stream as fast as alcohol without damage to the nutrients going through your digestive tract. This type of processing has minimum negative effect and maximum nutrient absorption. Doing this for a period of time, 15 to 30 days, makes a serious improvement to your health.

It is best to keep knifes and blenders away from fruits and vegetables, because the blades reduce life force energy from the food when it is cut. It is a form of processing, that isn't devastating but should be mentioned. The benefits of juicing fruits and vegetables outweigh the detriments to the processing of the juice, because of short circuiting the digestive tract, juice gets into the blood stream in about 15 minutes. The best juicer is the Gerson model because it doesn't "process" the vegetables, it squeezes it into a glass while sitting on your counter with a small 2 ton press. The cost though is 2500$ plus S&H. Regular juicer equipment sells for 200$+.

89.7 percent of Americans believe that they are eating a healthy diet meanwhile approximately 36 percent of all Americans are obese and 2/3 are overweight.

In the news it was found that meat passed off as beef in the U.K. was really horse meat. A recent analysis into several different fast food hamburgers found little meat and a lot of other stuff. According to GreenMedInfo, the study was to determine what exactly Americans are eating when they consume their 5 billion hamburgers annually. The burgers from 8 different fast food establishments were analyzed microscopically for tissue types. Their analysis found that water constituted about half of the weight of the burgers, with water content ranging from 37.7% to 62.4%. Meat was found to be as low as 2.1% in some cases, to the maximum of 14.8%. The balance contained questionable body parts. Even better, the meat in fast food hamburgers was found to have parasites and ammonia in it. The ammonia is used to kill the fecal matter of the animal in processing, and by the way ammonia is very toxic, even deadly. I speculate that the life force of a fast food hamburger is below zero.

On Youtube.com, I saw a hamburger and fries from the largest fast food chain window that sat on a shelf for 14 years without decomposing. At first glance it looked like it had been served that day. You can watch "Super Size Me" on Youtube.com to get a better understanding of the meaning of Life Force energy of food. The food tastes great but I can't eat it because it makes me sick with cramps.

Quick Solution for the food chapter is:

Drink non-toxic water,
Eat non-toxic food,
Eat high density nutrient meal replacement,
Eat and buy only organic everything,
Juice vegetables and fruit and eat them whole as well as salads,
Consume a few quality supplements.

Avoid food within ½ hour of drinking coffee, soda, alcohol, and smoking and never use a microwave! Avoid Aspartame, it is the feces of ecoli. There are over 6000 products now with this toxic aspartame on the market for your toxic consumption. Avoid GMO like the plague.

Cleanse your liver and kidneys, and say goodbye to health care costs. Disease can be resolved quickly with oxygen including Malaria and AIDS. But not all listed diseases are diseases. Sometimes they are symptoms of something else. I will try to address in chapter 8, but I propose that all illness can be traced back to the 5 elements of the Matrix and caused by inflammation as a result.

Water and Iodine

Our water is important because you can only live 4 or 5 days without it, and our water supply is being contaminated with fluoride, a toxic waste chemical used in the bleaching process in the production of aluminum manufacturing. Melon Andrew who was founder of ALCOA and currently is a major stockholder is in charge of public health services, advising municipalities to use fluoride, and encouraging regions to increase its concentration in the water supply. I believe a major conflict of interest? There is no science or ever was any science to prove that fluoride is good for your teeth or that it has any health benefit for human consumption. Ethical science has uncovered that it is responsible for dental fluorosis, making teeth brittle, fragile, yellowish, and causes pitting of the teeth. Anytime there has been a leak, the hazmut crews are called in and communities are evacuated under emergency conditions. That's what happened in Tennessee when a truck overturned. Fluoride burns through concrete and is as toxic as arsenic. They forget to report these events in the news. It was used in Nazi Jewish concentration camps to leave prisoners docile, dumb and obedient.

Manufacturing and baking is mostly done on municipal water supply, to ensure adequate volumes where these toxic chemicals are embedded. People absorb 4x the amount of fluoride or chlorine by showering in it, so just because you are off drinking tap water, you must change your shower filter to block out these chemicals. Watch, after your first shower how your hair and skin goes soft with less itch, and how easy you can put a comb through it. If you want nice hair, put filter on your shower.

Doctors report that, 17% of breast cancer is caused by estrogen mimickers like parabens, BPS, and BPA and the other of 83% is by low iodine. Vitamin B2 (Riboflavin) enhances utilization of iodine and it is best matched with Iodide for maximum bio availability. Lugols is a potent formulation of iodine at the pharmacy, but the Iodide formulation is better. There are 4 types of thyroid hormones T1, T2, T3, and T4, but T3 and T4 are the most important. Selenium enhances inactive T4 into active T3.

The fluoride and chlorine are also leaching out glycine and taurine amino acids out of your bodies and that is contributing to everyone who drinks municipal water, the formation of gallstones. I bet gallbladder removal is on the rise because of this.

Good Water

Well water is best from a natural supply. It has the highest chance of being fresh. Problems have been happening with rural communities who run off well water being able to light their water on fire coming out of the tap, because of fracking techniques being done miles away underground to extract natural gas below their properties. Bacteria and ecoli are really not a problem, they can be dealt with. Poison in the water is trickier and more expensive to remove and difficult to detect. Cities in France put h2o2 (food grade) to disinfect their water to keep it safe. It is 5000x more effective than fluoride/chlorine to disinfect the water supply, and this method delivers the water to the tap alive instead of dead with Life Force and continues to effectively take out diseased cells out of your body after you drink it, reducing health care costs. H2o2 is used throughout Europe!! Instead of dropping chlorine down dug and drilled wells to decontaminate them, it is healthier to drop h2o2 (food grade) down the well than poison which is the current practice. A liter down a drilled well and a gallon down a dug well, should be more than enough, but check with a book called One Minute Cure on the use of h2o2(food grade), and always use the municipal bacteria testing facility to be sure before you can trust the water for drinking.

Avoid using chlorine, bromine in your recreational pools, and hot tubs, and consider substituting with h2o2 (food grade) and consider adding ½ a cup to your baths to soak in. Diluted properly, it is an anti-disease agent on the skin and when it is absorbed, it promotes healthy cells and when you breathe in the steam off the water it is oxygen enriched and healing. A liter a week in a hot tub is about enough to sterilize and give life to its occupants. The vapor you breathe, will be healing to your lungs, to cuts, and to every cell it comes in contact with. Another excellent method to detox your hot tub water is using Ozone (O3) for sterilization.

GMO food contamination

Avoid bread, cereal, bran, corn, wheat, barley and anything with non-organic flour because it is GMO that contains a protein which turns to a pesticide poison in your gut, and is a major contributor to gluten intolerance because it is rich in that toxic protein your body has a hard time breaking down. It is believed that 50% of North Americans are now gluten intolerant because of GMO and it is in 80% of everything you eat, unless it is organic. Gluten free increases your chance of being GMO free but usually has other toxic substances contained.

There is such an outcry for this poison to be outlawed that millions are marching in protest around the world. Countries are doing their own scientific studies and burning thousands of acres of GMO crops in Hungary (Genetically Modified Food), Japan is banning the importation of anything that might have GMO contained from the US.

Organic USDA in my opinion goes too far in their strict rules for certification. In my opinion, it needs a second level because they unnecessarily drive up the cost of organic. As long as fruit and vegetables have the nutrients in them, with the soil preserved for future crops that should be perhaps the only qualification to qualify as a tier 2 organic level. It is the pesticides in the soil that are killing us. Backyard fruits and vegetables are as good, or even better than organic store bought because there is higher life force in the food absent of the destructive vibration of the truck drive from the crop to the store, along with the time it takes to get to your table.

So, backyard/organic grown fruits and vegetables are between 500-1000% when you look at the cross-section of nutrients that make up spinach. They are more nutritious than regular store bought fruits and vegetables that are not organic. You have to eat 8 salads from a restaurant or grocery store to match the equivalent nutrient value as 1 salad grown at home in your backyard or from an organic store. Weight gain and obesity to satisfy the average adult of their nutrient demand your body is calling for is a consequence. Organic is nothing special, and only means "regular"… "normal"…not poisonous". It takes years for mother-nature to return tortured soil back to natural conditions for normal harvest of nutrients. Monsanto is destroying the farmland of the world as well as the population that eats from the technology that comes out of their laboratories. The more your body has to eliminate poison or food substances your body doesn't recognize, the less vital your body and the higher your cholesterol levels will be along with a multitude of symptoms including a lowering of your IQ and your passion for life.

Alkaline Diets and energy

An alkaline diet will not make you alkaline. Alkalinity is a function of inflammation not diet. There is a thought that an alkaline diet will make you alkaline, not true. Only a diet that is bio available in source nutrients that are high in Life Force energy will get your blood to an alkaline 7.0 level. One measure of bioavailability is the ratio of nutrients to waste, the body must sort through. Waste is the non-useful form of food. Generally speaking, the closer to nature a nutrient gets, the more bio available it is, and the higher the life force contribution to the health of your cells to absorb and thrive. Anything that is not life sustaining is therefore a toxin, and that drains your body's energy trying to remove it, as opposed to gaining energy to enable you to thrive from natural sources from your food. An alkaline diet is typical of a diet that is alive and rich in nutrients but it is a mistake to say that an alkaline diet will make you alkaline and therefore is misleading and might limit the diversity of a full spectrum of beneficial foods that affect health.

25% of the population takes expensive statin medications. Statistics from the American Heart Association show that 75 million Americans currently suffer from heart disease, 20 million have diabetes and 57 million have pre-diabetes. I see similarities of the US population to the commercial cattle farming with cows falling over dead and obese on the day of slaughter by eating unnatural diets and caged up in unnatural settings. The trajectory is going up and is affecting younger and younger people every year. Over 90% can be remediated within 30 days. A person with 80% arterial blockage needing bypass surgery can be cleared in 15 days on a raw-food diet juicing and meal replacement. Arthritis eliminated in 15 days on a meal replacement, hypertension with 10 weekends of cleansing and flushing the liver. Cholesterol statin drugs gone following chapter 2 and 6 in 30 days. Cancer using chapter 2 with h2o2 food grade in 30 days and spike iodine if it is bone, or breast cancer. We can't guarantee results using the ideas in this book, but you should increase your probability of success by about a quadrillion% (give or take a billion) for success of the disease you are trying to remedy and every other ailment and pain you don't know you have at the same time.

Without inflammation being present in the arteries there would be no way for cholesterol to accumulate on the wall of the blood vessel to cause heart disease and strokes. When you chronically expose the blood vessels to injury by eating foods the human body was never designed to process, a condition occurs, called chronic inflammation, which is as harmful as acute inflammation is beneficial. The recommended mainstream diet that is low in fat and high in polyunsaturated fats and carbohydrates cause chronic inflammation leading to heart disease, stroke, diabetes and obesity.

An overload of highly processed carbohydrates of sugar, flour, and all the things made from them, and the excess consumption of omega-6 oils like soybean, corn and sunflower and canola oil that are found in many processed foods lead to inflammation of the arteries, looks like a brush has scrubbed it repeatedly. Foods loaded with sugar, HFCS (high fructose corn syrup), simple carbs, or processed with omega-6 oils for long shelf life creates small injuries daily. Blood sugar rises rapidly and in response, your pancreas secretes insulin whose primary purpose is to drive sugar into each cell where it is stored for energy, but if the cell is full, it doesn't need glucose and is rejected. When your cell rejects the extra glucose, blood sugar rises producing more insulin and glucose converts to stored fat. Blood sugar is controlled in a narrow range. Extra sugar molecules attach to an assortment of proteins that in turn injure the blood vessel wall just like sandpaper.

Not only do you have a problem with sweets but the chips and fries soaked in soybean oil, and processed foods are manufactured with omega-6 oils. Omega 6 is part of every cell membrane controlling what goes in and out of the cell and they must be in correct balance with Omega-3's. If the balance is out, the membrane produces inflammatory cytokines that cause inflammation which leads to obesity because of abnormal leptin levels. The North American diet has produced a massive imbalance between these 2 fats. The ratio of imbalance should be 3:1 for optimum health but they are as high as 15:1 and even as high as 30:1, Omega 6 to Omega 3. These foods create overloaded fat cells that excrete inflammatory chemicals caused by high blood sugar contributing to your heart disease, high blood pressure, diabetes and even Alzheimer's. The body was not designed to consume foods packed with sugars and soaked in omega-6 oils.

The solution is to consume carbohydrates that are complex such as organic fruits and vegetables. Use virgin olive oil or better coconut oil to cook with and avoid polyunsaturated oils.

Our World is Backwards where we Park on Driveways and We drive on Parkways?

Time to get aware

We need people to wake up because our government is choking off the supply of cleanses, supplements, high density nutrients and nutrition, to get and keep us healthy. Not only that, they are advising us to wear toxic suntan lotion and stay out of the healing rays of the sun we need to stay alive and vital. Our supply of oxygen h2o2 is being taken off the shelves in the health food stores, ozone, hyperbaric treatments are being restricted, and MMS to kill diseased cells is now illegal.

We saw Proposition 37 in California defeated when over 90% of the population wanted to have GMO labeled on food. The result of the official ballot was 43% within 60 days later in favor of labeling GMO food, and the bill was dead. What was the probability of that? Who is making the electronic machines where votes are cast into thin air, run by a computer program? I have seen court testimony where a computer programmer confesses to a judge that the programs he wrote for the equipment rigged elections. The non-electronic ballots are being counted privately because of, "security reasons, for your safety".

In the so-called evil empire of Venezuela, volunteers are growing organic gardens in the available lands of boulevards of their streets in their communities. For those that need a snack they can reach for an apple and can get a gallon of gas for less than a dollar. In the civilized country of the US, farmers producing raw organic milk that is safe and nutritious, the kind distributed 100 years ago are being thrown in jail along with the cocaine smugglers. A farmer in the US who lives on 100+ acre farm collecting rain water has been arrested and thrown in jail for doing so. I don't know which is worse, the people who made the law, the people who enforce this nonsense, or the prosecutors and judges that put them in jail? All should be placed in a mental institution for those who enforce insanity. There is a war going on with our food and water right now. There is a mandate being implemented that makes growing organic gardens in your front yards illegal. I suggest to home owners to start growing gardens where time and space permit in the boulevards and in your yard. Time for civil disobedience to stand up for our rights.

We can't guarantee health results, but you can be hiking up a mountain the day on the calendar your 6 oncologists tell you won't be around and telling you to, "get your affairs in order" with cancer throughout your body. You can use oxygen to get rid of disease along with the do's and don'ts of chapter 2 to get you thriving, all for the cost of a trip to Vegas? While you go on an anti-inflammatory diet of abundance from chapter 2, you need to stay away from inflammatory foods found in grocery stores.

Note: Oxygen only works on symptoms of inflammation like cancer and not the cause of disease unless that disease originates by a virus or bacteria, like AIDS.

One week of military spending, could wipe out suffering experienced worldwide from hunger

"Who controls the food and water supply controls the people,
who controls the energy can control whole continents;
who controls money can control the world."
Henry Kissinger

(seems he was right)

A BALANCED DIET IS A GLASS OF WINE IN EACH HAND

The elephants are hosting an animal conference. All the animals attend except one. Which animal does not attend? Answer next chapter.

Chapter 6

Toxic tissue - filters of the body and cleansing

Is the 4th most important element of the Health Matrix. Toxins in food and water kill life.

Toxic Loading vs Toxic Elimination

The challenge today is eliminating toxins faster than you acquire them. It is an equation. The body is efficient at eliminating toxins, but exposure to toxins has been ramping up in the recent decade. The efficiency of your liver has been declining with over burden of ever increasing toxic quantities and potency of substances in your food or water and along with that, there is rise in physical impedance of the liver's function with gallstones forming from biliary sludge. The bile thickens with a diet low in nutrients and high in chemical toxins like fluoride and chlorine leeching out cysteine and taurine amino acids, along with a general rise in inflammation, and disease. The elimination of nutrients from food for cellular repair together with the rise in toxins is the primary cause of inflammation in the body and the formation of gallstones in the liver and the inability of your body to remove dangerous cholesterol. The toxins then back up into the pancreas, which further result in blood sugar management problems and the rise in diabetes.

Intensification of radiation from wifi, smart meters, microwaves ovens, smart phones, television and electronic play stations, even remote car keys and remote garage door openers, your portable home phone is massive, cell tower intensifying radiation in 4G communicates to your cell phone now with 2 towers, all eroding the health of overworked immune systems while piling on more sources of inflammation but at the same time dissolving you of your ability to think from inside a mind floating in a sea of toxic electronic smog.

The trajectory of this problem is increasing with the introduction of GMO's, the intensification of toxins in vaccinations, the number and frequency of vaccinations, and chemtrails or geoengineering that is being sprayed as aerosols back and forth across our skies full of nano particulate of aluminum, barium, strontium, radiation in North America is having a devastating impact, stripping trees of their bark and resulting in respiratory problems, infection, inflammation, poor gut flora from a mountain of anti-biotics. Hospitals are plugged every time they spray over cities with neurotoxins and bacteria.

Filters

There are 3 main filters in your body the 2 kidneys, and the liver. The liver has 100,000 enzyme functions every second. The two other filters are the spleen and lymph nodes. The kidneys and the liver can be cleaned with multiple flushes and cleanses and the lymph nodes can be cleared with activities like jogging, rebounding on a trampoline or by massage moving the lymph nodes manually.

The Filters and Gout

Fish oil contributes to gout, so you could try primrose oil instead for your EFA's. When the liver fails to break down uric acid into separate carbon units, is part of the reason for gout and the need to clean that organ and your kidneys of stones and chemicals is important. It is essential to add selenium to your diet with iodine. Cherries prevent gout naturally. Just boiling a 3$ batch of organic parsley in a pot of 7 mugs of water for 20-25 minutes will clean your kidneys and get rid of pain after drinking just one mug of the parsley water by the next day. One pot of the broth will give you one mug a day for 5 days. Just drink a mug or two a day or if you have kidney problems. Being on dialysis will start to alleviate problems right away. Parsley tea is a cheap cleanse you should do regularly. This should raise energy levels for everyone who does this procedure, a day after you drink your first mug. You can substitute the water in your meal replacements with parsley tea from the fridge.

Glutathione is a powerful anti-oxidant and is about 100x more powerful than taking Vitamin C at bringing down inflammation throughout the body. I stir stir 2 scoops into a glass of water 1x a day and drink on an empty stomach, and this brings down inflammation and uric acid levels throughout your entire body. The most potent is injected via IV in a natural path's office. I hope to have a pail of it for about 40$ that could last a couple of months. Glutathione is great for diabetes, hepatitis and cancer and any disease where inflammation is involved. The anti-oxidant assists with cell apoptosis by taking out cells that are diseased or mutated and leaves the cells that can be repaired for the nutrients of meal replacement to heal. It's like a maid service and a handyman working together. There is a more powerful kidney cleanse that can be done to eliminate kidney disease below. I did them all for my kidney disease and continue to drink parsley water and take a powerful glutathione regularly for health maintenance. I hope to get this pail of glutathione in quantity for commercial sale.

Weight gain, hypertension, allergies and asthma

Significant excess weight around the belly is usually caused by a toxic liver plugged with parasites and gallstones. Being overweight is a symptom of inflammation, and inflammation is a precursor of many diseases like diabetes. A proper way to clean a liver is to first unplug it with a liver flush and then cleanse it of fats and toxins. Usually people with hypertension, allergies and asthma have excess weight to lose, so cleansing your liver should not only get rid of these symptoms but also give you the weight loss you are looking for. The excess weight usually reveals itself as a big belly when a sick liver is the cause. There are several additional benefits of cleansing as well, like raising your mood, your frequency, your passion for life, energy, IQ, endurance, mental illness, and countless benefits. I've seen 12 lbs lost on a single cleanse of someone who was 36kg/80 lbs. overweight. I've seen people with sick livers who were brought back to life that had a doctor say there is nothing wrong with their livers. It seems the doctor's tests are not sensitive enough to detect problems until it is too late.

SPLEEN The spleen filters old red blood cells and breaks them down and turns them into bile salts for excretion through the liver. An enlarged spleen is symptomatic of cancer somewhere present in the body.

GALLBLADDER/ LIVER So when we have bile salts float around in our blood, the liver filters these bile salts out of our system, collects them and sends them to the gallbladder. The gallbladder is a small organ that exists under the liver. A bladder is designed to hold liquid and the bile used to be called gall, that's why it's called a gall bladder. The gallbladder collects the liquid, extracts water soluble toxins and concentrates it. The end result is bile, a green, and strongly alkaline liquid. The bile acts as an emulsifier on the fat food solids to help aid digestion and it causes the large fat globules to break down into small droplets thereby creating a much greater surface area for the enzymes to work on digesting the fat in the digestion process.

The liver sends bile salts and waste down to the gallbladder. Two of the waste products are cholesterol and calcium. When there is an excess of calcium in the body, the liver extracts that from the blood and dumps it. The cholesterol appears when the liver produces more cholesterol than the digestive juices can liquefy, and the liver releases the excess into the gallbladder. These waste products are normally passed down with the bile when the gallbladder does its bile dump, and then on it goes down the tract for excretion. But sometimes they don't make it.

Sometimes these two waste products will crystalize and form gallstones. About 20% of gallstones are made of calcium, and about 80% are made of cholesterol. Gallstones can be as small like sand or as large as a golf ball. The older you get or if you have been ill, the better chance you have of having gallstones. People over 40, have a strong chance of having gallstones. Once you hit 50, men and women have them. When you get gallstones, you might get just get a large one, or you might get many various sizes. You might have hundreds of small ones, or even thousands of small ones. Normally, these will pass out of the gallbladder and pass out of the body. The problems occur when they get stuck.

When the gallstones get stuck, they cause problems of inflammation and improper functioning of the liver. Almost everyone with a serious disease or is over 40, or wants to lose weight should consider first a flush and then liver cleanses. An Epsom salt flush is rumored to go back as far as the Egyptians centuries ago. A flush is essential for optimum health for anyone. It's a little tricky to do but everything that is worthwhile, is. The key is killing the parasites before you do. Most everyone by the time they are 40 have adult parasites that are red in color, round in shape and as big as half the length and size of your pinky is round. These parasites block the flush of gallstones if they are not dead.

Kidney Stones

Chanca Piedra a supplement from Peru, has been used over time to dissolve calcium oxalate and uric acid crystals, the main ingredients of kidney stones.

Detoxification

Toxins are classified into two groups, those that are fat soluble and those that are water-soluble. Fat soluble toxins are released by the liver and secreted into the bile for excretion into the digestive tract. Water soluble toxins process through the kidneys and out through the urine. Maintaining this detoxification pathway by eliminating kidney stones, gallstones and biliary sludge is a prerequisite to any detoxification protocol.

Intestinal Health

Bile is responsible for many aspects of intestinal health. Bile neutralizes stomach acids, emulsifies fats, is a natural laxative and kills parasites and candida. Insufficient bile from gall bladder removal or gallstones can cause ulcers, malnutrition, constipation, lower immunity, contribute to low energy, depression, and allow parasitic and fungal to flourish. The liver, gall bladder and hepatic ducts can all suffer from accumulations of biliary sludge and gallstones. Bile, unable to pass into the duodenum can backwash into the liver and pancreas, causing alkaline burns. Traditional remedies for gallstones and biliary sludge involve drinking large quantities of Epsom salts, grapefruit juice and virgin olive oil in an attempt to cause contractions of the gallbladder resulting in a purge of biliary sludge, gallstones, and parasites. This kind of purge can be nauseous and does nothing to resolve the underlying cause of these accumulations of gallstones and sludge, just stones from the symptoms.

Step 1
Parasite Cleanse/ Basic Kidney Cleanse

The kidneys can be cleansed by boiling 3$ worth of organic parsley in a pot of water for 15 minutes. You drink a mug or 2 a day for a week for the kidney cleanse and then every month or two following for maintenance. If you have kidney disease you want to drink a mug everyday. It makes the pain in your kidneys go away quickly. Avoid GMO because it inflames your kidneys and leads to organ failure. Kidneys have a minor impact on your energy compared to an inflamed liver, but can be very draining if you are on dialysis.

It is important to do a parasite kill first using Extra Strength Clarkia drops while you do the kidney cleanse along with the parsley water cleanse. The parasites need to be killed before the flush, so when the pressure of the bile builds, following the liver flush protocol it will send them out as well, along with the gallstones. This procedure makes gallbladder removal and liver transplants and surgeries, other than trauma surgery, a thing of the past. Once the liver has been flushed you can begin to clean it with the liver cleanse instructions that follow Flush instructions. Weight loss will be off the charts and so will the euphoria of health following your efforts days and months following the series of cleanses as your body begins to function at optimum health.

The amount of Clarkia can be increased or decreased, depending on individual sensitivity. Signs that someone has taken too much is a headache. If you get a headache, decrease your amount. If you have no reaction to Clarkia, gradually increase the amount until you experience a headache, or until your dose reaches 60 drops total taken 3-5 times a day. Such high doses may be necessary for people with Cancer, AIDS, Diabetes, or people who have been unsuccessful in treating internal parasites or Candidiasis. For those patients don't hesitate to take Clarkia for months.

The procedure of kidney and liver cleanse is especially good for those that eat steak and red meat. There are a lot of parasites in that type of meat. It is best to eat meat from a 2 legged animal than a 4 legged one and always eat organic meat free of hormones, anti-biotics, arsenic that has a higher life-force free of chemicals and because the animals are not tortured. I noticed that non-organic chicken has a high fat content and low meat density that discourages me from buying food from a restaurant.

Step 2

Advanced Kidney Cleanse good for people on dialysis:

Hulda Clark pHD, ND, has a book published that has this herbal Kidney cleanse recipe in detail to help clean the kidneys from stones and eliminate pain and other urinary problems:

What you need for one Kidney cleanse:
65 gr. Hydrangea root
65 gr. Gravel root
65 gr. Marshmallow root
25 ml Goldenrod tincture 1 oz
200 ml Vegetable Glycerin
100 ml Black Cherry Concentrate
130 Ginger Capsules
42 Vitamin B6 Capsules (250mg)
42 Magnesium tablets (300mg)
126 Uva Ursi tablets
You need to buy 4 bunches of fresh parsley to start with.

How to do the Kidney cleanse:
Hydrangea root, Gravel root and Marshmallow root
Soak the root in 3 liters/quarts of cold tap water (avoid metal containers)
After 4 hours heat to boil, add 1/2 of the Black Cherry Concentrate.
Simmer for 20 minutes
Drink 1/4 cup 2 oz, as soon as it is cool enough
Pour the rest through a strainer into a sterile pint jar (glass) and several freezable containers. Refrigerate the glass jar, freeze the rest.
Store the roots in the freezer.
When your supply runs low, boil them again with other half of Black cherry concentrate but only with 2 liters/quarts of pure water and simmer only for 10 minutes
Do this a 3rd time if you run low on supply (use only 1.5 l/qt water)
Boil the fresh parsley, after rinsing, in 1 liter/qt of water for 3 minutes.
Drink 60 ml when cool enough, 2 oz
Refrigerate one half and freeze the other half. Throw away the parsley. Buy more fresh parsley when your supply runs low and do it again.

Note: Both the herbal tea and the parsley water can easily spoil within a week. The lengthen life just drop in 3 or 4 drops of Hydrogen Peroxide (food grade about 7$ for a year's supply at the health food store) in container and stir.

Step 3
About the Epsom Salt Liver Flush for gallstones and parasites

The Epsom salt liver flush has been around for thousands of years. It is a flush protocol made famous by Hulda Clark, a naturalpathic doctor. Epsom Salt is used to open your tubules in your gallbladder and the oil slams out your gallstones under pressure for excretion. To help unplug the liver Extra strength Clarkia is sold off the internet at www.Clarkia. biz to kill parasites before the flush. Parasites cause cravings for food often containing sugar. Below is how to get rid of the parasites along with gallstones to get you liver back to functioning properly. Liver cleanse should be followed once blockages are removed.

Phosphatidyl Choline capsules should be taken 10 days prior to your flush dosed at 800-1000 mg per day to thin out bile along with the Extra Strength Clarkia drops for the parasites. This helps reduce nausea. The nausea experience is from blockage on flush day from parasites.

Flushing the liver of gallstones dramatically improves digestion, physically unblocks the liver to get it to functioning which is the foundation of health. Following, you can expect your allergies to disappear, with each flush you do. It also eliminates shoulder, upper arm, and upper back pain. You have more energy and an increased sense of well being. Flushing the liver bile ducts is the most powerful cleanse procedure that you can do to improve your body's health. But do the parasite procedure first and take extra strength Clarkia 20 drops 3x/day for 7-10 days in a glass of water and for best results should follow the kidney cleanse. Boil a clump of organic parsley in a pot of water of 7-9 mugs and boil for 15 minutes and throw out the parsley. Pour remaining water into a jug and drink one mug a day for about 7 days while you are killing the parasites.

It is the job of the liver to make bile, 1 to 1½ liters/quarts in a day! The liver is full of tubes (biliary tubing), intrahepatic bile ducts, that deliver the bile to one large tube the common bile duct. The gallbladder is attached to the common bile duct and acts as a storage reservoir. Eating fat or protein triggers the gallbladder to squeeze itself empty after about twenty minutes, and the stored bile finishes its trip down the common bile duct to the intestine.

For many persons, including children, the biliary tubing is choked with gallstones. Some develop allergies or hives but others have no symptoms. When the gallbladder is scanned or X-rayed nothing is seen. Typically, they are not in the gallbladder. Most are too small and not calcified, a prerequisite for visibility on X-ray. There are over half a dozen varieties of gallstones, most of which have cholesterol crystals in them. They can be black, red, white, green or tan colored.

The green ones get their color from being coated with bile. Other stones are composites, made of many smaller ones. At the center of each stone is found bacteria, suggesting that a dead bit of parasite might have started the stone forming.

As the stones grow and become more numerous the back pressure on the liver causes it to make less bile. It is also thought to slow the flow of lymphatic fluid. With gallstones in the way, less cholesterol leaves the body, and cholesterol levels rise. Gallstones are porous, and can pick up bacteria, cysts, viruses and parasites that are passing through the liver. In this way pockets of infection are formed, forever supplying the body with fresh bacteria. No stomach infection such as ulcers or intestinal bloating can be cured without removing gallstones from the liver.

Flush Day

Reminder: You can't clean a liver with living parasites in it, but you won't get many stones, and you will feel quite sick. Zap daily the week before and complete the parasite killing program before attempting a liver cleanse. If you are on the maintenance parasite program, you are always ready to do the liver flush.

Doing the kidney cleanse before flushing the liver is recommended. You want your kidneys, bladder and urinary tract in top working condition so they can efficiently remove any undesirable substances absorbed from the intestine as the bile is being excreted.

Ingredients

Epsom salts ¾ tablespoon per glass of 6 oz of water. You will need 4 glasses of salt water in total.

Extra Virgin Olive oil 1/2 (half cup) 4 oz + 2 fresh grapefruits, squeezed into fill 2/3 cup 6 oz to mix with the oil = 10 oz. total of oil and grapefruit juice.

Total = 4 + 1.

Ornithine amino acid 5 to 7 tablets ready for bedtime, to be sure you can sleep and helps to relax the liver to open. Don't skip this or you may throw up. The nausea is caused by blockage and the first flush will be the hardest to get things moving and unplugged. I would suggest using extra virgin olive oil, and try 3 oz on your first attempt and wait 10-14 days between cleanses to allow your body to regroup before going to maximum strength 4 oz. of oil. Oil is the active ingredient for the flush, everything works around this center point. Taking the oil is what causes the nausea.

Choose a weekend for the flush, since you will be able to rest the next day. Take no medicines, vitamins or pills that you can do without, they could prevent success. Stop the parasite and kidney program and kidney the day before. Eat a no-fat breakfast and lunch such as cooked oatmeal, fruit, fruit juice, or honey but no butter or milk. This allows the bile to build up and build pressure in the liver. Higher pressure pushes out more stones.

Sequence:

2:00 PM. Do not eat or drink after 2 o'clock. If you break this rule you could feel quite ill later.

6:00 PM. Drink one serving ¾ cup of the water with epsom salts. You may add 1/8 tsp. Vitamin C powder to improve the taste if you want. You may also drink a few mouthfuls of water afterwards or rinse your mouth.

8:00 PM. Repeat by drinking another cup of Epsom salts/ water mix. You haven't eaten since two o'clock, but you won't feel hungry. The timing is critical for success.

9:00 PM. Take 5-7 ornithine capsules with the first sips to make sure you will sleep through the night. Take 8 if you suffer from insomnia.

9:45 PM. Pour 1/2 (half) cup of olive oil into a glass.
Or just 3oz if you want to build up to full strength for the next cleanse 2 weeks later.
Grapefruit is squeezed by hand into the measuring cup. Remove pulp with fork. You should have ¾ of a cup (three fourths/6 oz) of grapefruit juice and mix this vigorously with the 3 or 4oz of Extra Virgin oil depending on your courage to do partial strength or full strength. Total 9-10 oz.

10:00 PM. Drink the oil/ grapefruit potion you have mixed.
Lie down immediately. You might fail to get stones out if you don't. The sooner you lie down the more stones you will get out. As soon as the drink is down walk to your bed and lie down flat on your back with your head up high on the pillow. Try to think about what is happening in the liver. Try to keep perfectly still for at least 20 minutes. You may feel a train of stones traveling along the bile ducts like marbles. There is no pain because the bile duct valves are open, thanks to the Epsom salts.

Next Morning

Take your third dose of Epsom salts/6 oz water mix in a glass when you wake up. If you have indigestion or nausea wait until it is gone before drinking more Epsom salts. You may go back to bed. Don't take this morning mixture before 6:00 am.

8:00am (2 hours later), take your fourth and last mixture of Epsom salts/ 6oz water in a glass and you may go back to bed again.

10:00am After 2 More Hours you may eat but gently.
Start with fruit juice. Half an hour later eat fruit. One hour later you may eat regular food but keep it light. By supper you should feel recovered.

Expect diarrhea in the morning. Look for gallstones in the toilet. Look for the green kind since this is proof that they are genuine gallstones, not food residue. Only bile from the liver is pea green. Gallstones float because of the cholesterol inside. Count them all roughly, whether tan or green.

You will need to total 2000 stones before the liver is clean enough to rid you of allergies, bursitis or upper back pain permanently. The first cleanse may rid you of them for a few days, but as the stones from the rear travel onward, they give you the same symptoms again. You may repeat cleanses at two week intervals. Never cleanse or flush when you are ill. Sometimes the bile ducts are full of cholesterol crystals that did not form into round stones. They appear as chaff floating on top of the toilet bowl water. It may be tan colored, harboring millions of tiny white crystals. Cleansing this chaff is just as important as purging stones. How safe is the liver cleanse? It is very safe for many persons in their seventies and eighties. It can make you feel quite ill for one or two days afterwards, although in every one of these cases the maintenance parasite program had been neglected. This is why the instructions direct you to complete the parasite and kidney cleanse program first.

CONGRATULATIONS

You have taken out your gallstones without surgery! The origin of this cleanse was invented thousands, of years ago by the Egyptians! You must repeat Epsom Salt flush 2 weeks later to get rid of eggs of the parasites and remaining stones. You can repeat again in 2 more weeks for more effect but not sooner. Keep taking the 60 drops of Clarkia to kill parasites between cleanses.

Step 4
IsaCleanse, Cleanse for Life

Once the epsom salt flush is done, it's great to do the IsaCleanse for deep cellular cleansing for chemicals and fats stored in the liver and down stream through the digestive tract. This will have profound effect on the health of your liver and for weight loss and will help with allergies, chemical sensitivities, asthma hypertension and even LDL/ HDL cholesterol levels.

I used Isacleanse from Isagenix.com and took 2 scoops of the powder into a glass of water spread out 4x/day for two days 48-54 hours no food, vitamins and eliminating any drugs that are not deemed necessary by your doctor. When you are cleansing you should drink 2-3 oz. of water every 15 minutes. If you get a headache, that is a reminder to drink water more frequently. Repeat every 7-14 days with this cleanse, until there is no more improvement or unhealthy weight loss. The cleanse removes toxins and fats that get the liver functioning at ultimate health. The cleanse maintenance should be done every 6 months. If you drink alcohol regularly, perhaps once every 3 months would be better.

Follow cleanses with meal replacement which is high in nutrient density. I believe that the amount of nutrients in a blended glass of water is equivalent of 10 meals of nutrients per scoop with only 250 calories. The most you should take is 4 scoops (100 grams of protein) of meal replacement a day spread throughout the day because too much protein can be hard on the kidneys. Like the kidney and liver cleanses, taking the high density nutrition is a major source of healthy weight loss, by lowering leptin, visceral fat and inflammation. In the case of someone getting out of a hospital bed with atrophy, meal replacement protein shakes are a major source of healthy weight gain. It doubles the speed of recovery from surgery and reduces pain and inflammation following surgery significantly. You should supplement protein shakes with organic fruits and vegetables, and avoid GMO's, they are inflammatory to your organs we have just tried to clear and clean. Meal replacement is different than protein shakes, in that it has more vitamins and minerals.

Step 5

There is GALLSTONE FLUSH that is an easy method to get rid of gallstones without using Epsom salts and oil. The formula comes as a suppository, 10 in a box and are good for people who have had their gallbladders removed. A must have for the all the sick and elderly who can't handle the nausea associated with the epsom salt cleanse. With gallstones removed you have a profound improvement in health. The drawback is that it costs more. The formula incorporates glycine, taurine, phosphatidyl choline (pc) and chanca piedra as the main ingredient. The formation of gallstones is partly caused by a lack of glycine and taurine from drinking and bathing in municipal water. The chanca piedra breaks the stones up and phosphatidyl choline thins out the bile. Magnesium can help to soften stones.

Step 6

Royal Flush

Works by removing the crust build up on the wall of the digestive track of foreign substances. The benefit of the removal exposes more surface area of the digestive tract to allow for more absorption of nutrients. It uses bentonite that expands to change the shape of the digestive tract to force the non-malleable substances to break free for excretion.

Step 7

Chelation, there are several types, mostly for heavy metal removal done by intravenous in a doctors office. See chapter 8.

Step 8

There is another kidney cleanse using cantaloupe. After cleaning the skin you cut an entire cantaloupe including the skin into strips and push through a blender and drink the mash. Following eating this mash, your urine will be cloudy for a day where it is discharging dead cells as dead protein. It is another cleanse you should try but I didn't find it as effective as parsley tea.

Step 9

Borax cleanse and Morgellons

The cleanse is best done after cleaning your kidneys and liver because Borax is toxic and can accumulate, by putting 1/8th teaspoon of boron ingredient found in Borax laundry detergent into a liter/ quart of water and sipping it throughout the day. Spreading out the consumption over the course of a day is necessary. You do this for 4 days on and 3 days off for 2 cycles but for Morgellons daily for weeks is necessary. The noticeable effects are an increase of energy, a decrease in arthritis symptoms, an improvement of eyesight, an increase in sex drive, balancing of hormones, elimination of hot flashes, increase in testosterone availability for males, and an increase of estrogen. Borax kills yeast that causes vaginal infections, lowers plasma lipid levels and helps with removal of cholesterol, increases brain and cognitive functions, short term memory, and concentration. It is good for killing parasites, candida, allergies, helps with aging, osteoporosis (by lowering inflammation), and menopause symptoms. Boron is deficient in soil, produce and pastures, so it is good for eliminating arthritis in horses and farm animals and your pets. It is has a positive effect on the magnesium and phosphorous minerals in your body. These 2 elements are in short supply from commercial farming that is not respecting the aged old practice of crop rotation and the use of pesticides killing the soil.

The cleanses used in conjunction with one another should have profound effects on your body's performance. This is just a short list of benefits you should experience.

The Borax cleanse should be considered last of the cleanses. There is a caution for people with kidney problems. Borax has a molecular weight of 5 on the periodic table of elements and is eliminated through the urine and it can be accumulated in the body. Morgellons disease seems to be another planted bug from Plum Island off Lymes Connecticut courtesy of our Authorities. Borax cleanse worked to kill Morgellons disease for those who have it and was used in conjunction with h2o2. Morgellons is a new disease that is emerging on the horizon and is thought to come from the combination of vaccinations, GMO's and chemtrails. (see chapter 8)

Answer from chapter 5:
The zebra. The zebra is in the refrigerator. You just put him in there. This is a test of your memory.

Chapter 7

Frequency

Vibration/ Mood/ Sense of Euphoria/ Attitude/ Gratitude is the best attitude.

"If you want to find the secrets of the universe, think in terms of energy, frequency and vibration." Nikola Tesla

If you are going on a road trip across the country, or you want to start an exercise program, have a surgery, or are considering physiotherapy without first changing your oil and being certain your filters are clean, you are divorcing intellect from wisdom.

With health, ask yourself:

How does it get better?
What is it going to take?
What else is possible?
What's right about this, I'm not getting?

Everything good begins with health. With the extra energy you achieve with new health, you will then want to direct it towards setting more goals.

Practice:

- Letting go of negative thoughts as they arrive by being still and visualize releasing. Grounded to the earth and or using Solfeggio frequencies off Youtube.com is intensely calming to release.

- The goals you visualize need to be in alignment with helping people. Law of attraction.
- Try to be in alignment with your talents and gifts. A talent could be an ability to make someone or people feel good. It helps if can find your purpose in life, everyone has one. Some cultures call this Dharma.
- Removing doubt gets you to where you are going sooner. You are pure potential. Practice confidence.
- Embrace success no matter how small, and let go of failures as strictly lessons.
- Give freely of yourself and this opens the door of receiving.
- Be open and follow the path of least effort absent of structure through harmony and synergy.
- Try detaching from the prison of past hurts and conditioning that limits you and your worthiness of success. You are worthy.
- What's true makes you feel lighter and a lie makes you feel heavier.
- Have good intentions with your actions and thoughts through your efforts, embrace "Karma".

Frequency is the 5th most important element in the matrix to affect your health. It is a minor element to affect your pH but is important because its subtle influence can affect you profoundly over time. Apathy, stress and fear are the enemy of health, while gratitude is the best attitude. You need the 4 elements in peak performance or balance to have a good influence on your frequency, but you need a good frequency to maintain the 4 elements of your health over time.

The body is an instrument that when it is not operating properly will let you down emotionally, and rarely the opposite. It is not hard to comprehend how devastating our food and water and consumer products have become. The normal was of 100 years ago when 1 in 100,000 kids had autism and now the statistic is 1 in 50, but to some extent, for everyone who decide to take a vaccination today it is 100%. With so many toxins in our body, it makes me believe that disease does not come from your head.

Love of yourself, someone, and or something are ways you can use to achieve your high frequency in the present, borrowing inspiration from the past to dream about pleasant times ahead for the future. You will find a higher vibration if you don't already have one with thoughts of desire. Happiness is the recipe for success found first through health, not money. Being a member of a yacht club for years, the happiest people I saw were people in the smallest boats with a fishing rod and a cooler. If you are unhappy without money you will be unhappy with it.

I've experienced both. The only thing you experience by having abundance is you get to enjoy more freedom and more respect of others, and shallow admiring attractive singles. My thoughts about that are, that I don't need anyone's respect because I have my own, shallow singles I could live without because the person that taught me the most from the heart was someone who lived on welfare and didn't care about money and possessions. LET GO.

Love vs Fear

The human mind only has two ways to think. One is in love and the other is fear. If you are angry or jealous you are in fear. Passion is the highest frequency and apathy is the lowest. Instead of complaining or filing a complaint, try referring to it as problem recognition. Complaining and complaints are the lowest form of frequency along with apathy, but at least with complaining it can be viewed as a form of passion. Someone who is complaining from anger, rage or someone who is threatening is actually in fear. To prove it, listen to what they say, stay attentive and then sympathize with the problem they have just unloaded, and then repeat their story as best you can, and watch the rage dissipate moving from a state of fear closer to love, closer to neutral, closer to laughter. To summarize engage the enraged, acknowledge with sympathy, and prove concern by repeating their story in your own words. Someone who can reiterate a complaint proves that you were listening, comprehended, and therefore are capable of fixing the problem and or improving the situation which brought on the rage. The fear of the enraged is you can't, you don't care, you wont, or you are incapable or resolving their problem.

Attention kids: adults are really children in adult bodies but living with more responsibilities. If you ever get mad at someone, look at how you react differently if you treat that person as if they are 8 years old when you are frustrated. A fun game I played with the kids is that I would pretend to be the child and they would pretend to be the adults. That was the most fun

I had. Some adults are incapable of evolving from a child in some areas and excel in others. I had some adults who believed that my condition of being in a wheelchair was in my head, and that I could have stood up out of it anytime I wanted. We agree to disagree. But in this case they were the child, despite being adult.

I had doctors asking me to leave their office as I was explaining my symptoms as I was declining with symptoms of deteriorating health into a wheelchair. I didn't judge them I just sympathized with them thinking back. They are practicing health care without understanding the subject. They are unfortunate victims of a system of control that doesn't serve the purpose of the community but the interests of corporations that have authority. Authority is dangerous. I learned that Authority has a monopoly on health care and makes its own laws that serve its own interests. Most doctors haven't connected the dots on health to see health with any kind of clarity. Authority keeps the dots apart so the won't see the picture using compartmentalization and the general public is put in a trance-like state with big words and complex ideas but they don't understand health. Humanity has been programmed from the time a child is born to accept what their parents believe is real, reinforced by schools, churches, family into a prison cell of conformity. George Orwell said, "if you control history, you control the present".

Moving onto Solutions

Embrace the do's don'ts list in chapter 2 as best you can on your budget to embrace health. For those who can't afford the extras on these lists, get as much sunshine on your skin as you can safely expose, connect your skin to the earth as much as you can, avoid wearing non-organic sunscreen, avoid sunglasses as much as possible, find spring water and avoid municipal water, and express positive affirmations each morning and ask for protection and help from your angels each day. Call upon your angel for help.

There are angels here for everyone on earth to heal you now. There are more of us than there are of them. All you have to do embrace health for 30 days and ask for help from your angels. Meet them half way, perhaps all you need is 15 days to start seeing the results you want to start believing? For the miracle of health to emerge ask for their help, show them you want help. Make it a priority to bring your body out of obesity, out of inflammation, out of disease, off medication, out of hopelessness. For those that see the results, share your success with others!

For those of you with disease discover h2o2 hydrogen peroxide food grade 29 or 35% from a health food store for 7$ for a year's supply (refrigerate) for you and your extended family They have instructions or you can buy One Minute Cure handbook for directions is best.

We need the help of Dr. Shoemaker to come forward to help us with the cause and cure of autoimmune, and his latest ideas emerging about MS, Lymes and chronic Lymes.

You need to do 5 things to achieve this or move in this direction significantly.

5 Basic steps:
Flush your liver with Dr. Hulda Clark method of gallstones and parasites I hope to bring forward a suppository method.

Clean your liver I like the Isacleanse by Isagenix.com for toxins and fats.

Meal replacement 2x/day in a glass of parsley water.

Iodine I think a triple dose a day for the first 6 months would be best and check with your doctor regularly as your thyroid becomes active again. I hope to bring forward a superior product.

Juicing Organic vegetables and fruits daily 12-16 oz.

Hormones if you are over 40, DHEA for men 50 mg/day and Progesterone for women each day postmenopausal or the last 15 days of your cycle. It's best to check with a Bio Identical Hormone specialist first.

Compassion is the basis for Buddhism. If you dream a goal or an outcome with passion, try to avoid those that get in the way. There is always a critic in the crowd. So, love is the highest frequency, fall in love with someone or something. Manifest what you love, not what your fear. If you are in a wheelchair, and you are in a hospital with cancer, think about the sailboat you are going to sail on when you get out. Borrow inspiration from the past and bring it into the future to get out of the low frequency of the now. Let go of regret they are just lessons and you hope not to repeat too many.

Recovery for me was a ladder as high as a mountain that involved 3 steps forward and 2 steps back. No matter how bad your situation, there is someone who is worse off, seemed to be my relief valve. My experience as an invalid could have been shortened to months from years with what I learned and could have been completely avoided with what I know now. But I have no regrets just lessons. What I learned was to look at things in a different way. It is not so much about what is wrong, your focus should be more on what isn't right, because whatever is wrong with you can be reversed. What is wrong with you is a mirror image of what is right. When you reverse inflammation there could be a 50% improvement in your disease, success that parallels improvement throughout your whole body should also equal to 50%. What you have done is increased your level of health, and by doing that you have raised all of the ships with it.

Fear: False Evidence Appearing Real

There are areas you could look at that can help you follow a path of least resistance to achieve positive attitude. But first you first need to realize that the human mind only has 2 states of being. One is in fear with worry and one is love without worry. The word love can be confusing but it is synonymous with passion, having profound interest or curiosity. The antonym of passion is apathy. You are born perfect so don't be hard on yourself, others can do it for you! If you find you are unfilled in your life and a feeling of apathy comes over, you can change this quickly by using the power of now. Get out to a park and feed some chipmunks, or lace up a pair of roller blades, or go to a park and watch children playing, or do yoga, meditate or buy a book to learn. Take time to be still and be calm, breathe deeply in through your nose and fill your chest. Calm is a place from where genius comes. BREATHE.

I would like to apologize to anyone I have not offended. Please be patient. I will get to you shortly.

Opinions are different than mine about the subject of Frequency. It is the abstract element of our lives, but one thing is in common for all, if you are not motivated by love, to live with healthy weight, or can find a passion, or you are motivated by materials things out of ego, you will never find true happiness. You will only find true happiness through love and the Beatles sang the song "Money can't buy you love", but it helps. The fact that you are reading this book is an indication of a curiosity of achieving a passion or enhancing it through health. Avoid drifting into bad habits of starvation diets, drinking alcohol, smoking, and avoid people that have bad habits that are unhealthy. These people usually lack a passion in their lives, sometimes damage done by critics and hard circumstances throughout their lives.

Passion vs Apathy

People are not created equal and it is wrong to assume that they are. I think a new system that evaluates people like they do in golf with handicaps would be a good idea. If kids could be evaluated and assessed a handicap early, a handicap of 2-4$ an hour could be supplemented continuously year to year perhaps for life. The person washing the dishes is just as important as the server, the cook, the owner, right? The dishwasher deserves a holiday, a place to live, and a night out a week. My point is that the person who does the dishes deserves self esteem. So if they are stuck washing dishes or stuck in a menial job for the rest of their lives and don't have the aptitude to own the restaurant, or to become a doctor, we need to maintain their dignity while they are a child before it's destroyed. The fragile teenager is just as human and we could stop driving teenagers into the streets with low self esteem as if they are someone inferior unworthy of self esteem. These people were the ones most to inspire me. Be mindful of the wants of Ego, and consider the needs of others. Needs matter and are part of being human. Know that wants can be selfish. Want is a lust and love is a need. CONSIDERATION.

Humans are electromagnetic beings with 7 chakras energy points and a torus field around your body that radiates out up to 50 feet. Your frequency of your body actually goes up as you detoxify and nourish your cells. The Torus is the form that the flow of energy takes at every scale of existence. The torus is the magnetic energy field around the earth, around a cell, around you, and around the entire universe. It is perfect in shape and flows through your chakras. The Torus is balanced, self regulating and always whole. When your torus grows, your problems seem to shrink and when that happens, it has been mathematically proven to increase your bliss. Priorities change from material things and living in Ego, to achieving higher levels of health, so people enjoy life at this level of evolvement and talk about ideas instead of things. Society and TV equate happiness to things and how much you own, but true happiness is the euphoria of health and acceptance of others and your situation as it is without fear or judgment, it's just a journey. What you have or what you own is not who you are. It's not where you're from but where you are going. What you see is what you believe. What you feel is what is. Anything else limits potential if you are stuck in belief. Madness is doing the same thing over and over and expecting different results. SURRENDER.

The Golden Mean Ratio generates life, it is self organizing. For waves of energy to meet, powers of 2 called "octive waves" are destructive. Golden mean waves when they meet leaves the energy intact after waves have interacted. The golden mean ratio is expressed as 0.6181 and it can both be added and multiplied, it is the reason life exists and has divine properties. It is the solution to compression and therefore the solution to constructive interference. It is the solution to physics, spirituality and bliss. Fractal is life and infinite in its form of perfect compression. Spirituality is perfect when you can add and multiply the wave length and the wave velocity. Perception, bliss and enlightenment gives you a peak experience when the magnetic map of aura looks like a rose. The "flower of life" is the "Lotus" opened up wide and its diagrams are on the walls of the great pyramids. Charge distribution efficiency equals life. It is the physics of Feng Shui. Another way put, is that fractality is geometry of perfect distribution of life, therefore is life itself. THINK.

Human chakras appear like fiery spinning suns spinning clockwise in the body and are connected to other chakras through the aura spin that runs vertically and is located at the back of each chakra. The diagram depicts the traditional 7 chakras that make up your energy field on a basic level. These chakras are what Reiki healing and crystal healing focus on. Both methods had profound beneficial affects on my journey of healing on the etheric level by profound practitioners.

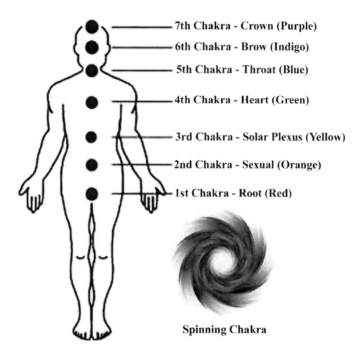

7th Chakra - Crown (Purple)
6th Chakra - Brow (Indigo)
5th Chakra - Throat (Blue)
4th Chakra - Heart (Green)
3rd Chakra - Solar Plexus (Yellow)
2nd Chakra - Sexual (Orange)
1st Chakra - Root (Red)

Spinning Chakra

The Seven Chakras:

THE BASE

Is known as the base or root chakra. It is situated at the base of the spine and is closely aligned to your earthly issues, like money, safety, shelter, survival, and the physical body. Practicing yoga, light exercise, and accupuncture help keeps the energy flowing by opening up meridian points. It is associated with the color red. Properly aligned you can tap into wisdom. It is the element of earth.

SACRAL

Is the second chakra associated with the color orange and with water. It is located 2 inches below the naval and is associated with desires, creativity, emotions and sexuality. To balance, practice yoga, nurture yourself, exercising and dancing help. This is the area where healers get their power.

SOLAR PLEXES

Is the third associated with fire and the color yellow. It represents vitality, power, self esteem and confidence. It is located just below the rib cage. It is associated with inner feeling and is a major reception area.

HEART

It is associated with the color green and the air element. It is parallel to the heart and in the center associated with compassion, love, harmony, healing and relationships. This is a chakra that needs extra healing energy by practicing forgiveness, and by loving yourself and others help you to become more in tune with spirit. This chakra connects mind, body and soul.

THROAT

It is associated with light blue and sound. It is located in the throat area where communication, creativity, sound and the ability of clairaudience comes from. Singers, speakers and actors have developed throat chakras. Singing and toning develop this area and the inspiration of creativity.

THIRD EYE

Is associated with indigo and with the element of light. Is the clairvoyance inner seeing, associated with intuition, and linked to higher levels of consciousness. Located on the lower center part of your forehead between your eyes.

CROWN (7th)

Is associated with the color violet and the element of thought. It is associated with your link to the center of the universe, your higher consciousness. It is the receiver of light and disperses energy throughout your aura for total well being. It will allow you to tap into the deepest sources of wisdom.

I believe that the subject of the etheric healing principles is beyond the realm of most readers that are having a hard time believing that a cure could exist outside the practice of the current medical system in the 3D. The cure for everything has been found, it's not 100% but it's close. There was nothing I couldn't find a cure for and that's all I did. I hear of healing chambers technology that is here currently that can be released to the public, once it is safe to do so. I believe that there are better ways to heal still to reveal themselves and I believe that there isn't a cure that exists within the current health care system or ever has been one. I am living proof of that and the other success stories I have met.

The earth actually gives off healing energy when you connect to it without rubber soled footwear. The boost in energy, I estimate is about 1% Life Force added, but it takes about an hour of physical connection. This is ambiguous but you can learn more about Life Force energy on the science of Fractality, that brings Einstein's theory on the Unified Field together of how gravity, rainbows, black holes, and bliss is measured mathematically.

Humans come from consciousness which is thought. Consciousness is a form of energy when its frequency is slowed down, then becomes light. When the light frequency is slowed down, it becomes a lower expression of energy in a lower dimension. As that energy slows down it then becomes human form. Humans come from consciousness to experience or live in the third dimension. When you die you go back to the light in a higher dimension. That's why people who come back from a near death experience briefly see the white light and feel euphoric absent of pain. People who die generally are feeling pain first before they go to or see the light. My mother was one of those that witnessed this phenomenon and so have many others I have met. When you see the light, is when your soul is actually going to a higher dimension as your soul is folding in perfect compression absent of your body that remains in the 3rd dimension and the pain is released as you separate to the higher frequency of light energy of where you came from into the 5th. If you follow through on your journey of death to the white light, you determine your next life experience before you reincarnate as a baby with a birth date as the energy you will hold and use and experience into your next life without any memory of your previous life. Only your soul remembers your previous lives and is your guide in the new life. You can only connect to your soul by meditation, yoga, health, numerology, astrology, palmistry absent of fear and interference from the 4th (that doesn't have your best interests at heart). Angels exist in the 5th and higher dimensions of love. This information is not important, but is here in case you wanted to know.

The science of numerology has profound significance like that of astrology. The universe works in mysterious ways that are not sinister. Choice always remains yours and abundance will flow provided it is not selfish, but be mindful because karma enters into the equation. The universe does not tolerate hurting another. Be open and embrace your fears of culture and experience with trust. You can read more about the Tetrahedron, the Mercaba, and The Ancient Secrets of the Flower of Life by Drunvalo Melchizedek.

The great thing about a rumor is you get to learn so much about yourself you didn't know

Everything in the universe is energy. All energy moves in a wave. All waves vibrate at a frequency. Frequency is a thumbprint of someone's love energy measurable on a scale. Frequency can be summed up as how much love a wave is holding. Love is the highest frequency. Fear, frustration, rage and jealousy are the lowest frequencies. Things get better exponentially when you are emitting a high frequency of love. The frequency you emit will attract a like frequencies, it is how you manifest using the accepted Law of Attraction provided that what you are attracting is in your soul's alignment. With the science of the quickening along with the subject of the Mayan calendar together with the rising of the earth's frequency from 7.8 hertz to 13.8 hertz this decade, manifestations will come quicker. If you are in a high frequency you will attract good things and if you are in a low frequency you will attract bad things. So finding ways to stay or get into a positive frame of mind will help you while you are healing. Manifest what you love, not what you fear. You can find more on the subject in the book "Ultimate Power, by Linda West" on Amazon.

The earth is not flat. Authority knew that back 500 years ago, and that carbon dates the age of propaganda. The ascension will happen in the next 10 years currently marked scientifically by the pole shift and the rising of the earth's frequency from 7.8 Hz to 13.8 Hz. The change will be subtle and it is happening now in step with the awakening of people. People are starting to become aware of corruption and soon when the system crashes the reward is free energy, debt forgiveness in a world absent of illness. The awakening is the first step, the second step is embracing health, the third step then is demanding change and the forth step is to surrender to a great future for all absent of fear. You don't need to believe, you need to observe and be open and watch for the signs of change, but you need to be healthy to participate. Your body has voltage and is electrical in nature.

"Evil is live" spelled backwards.

Life is like a wave you ride to the beach but over a lifetime. The beach is your retirement, the bigger your wave the more money you can use in your retirement if you can ride it in. If you are healthy you can stay on that wave and retirement is good, but when your health fails that wave can come crashing down. Getting back on your board to catch the next wave can be hard without a health system to get you back up.

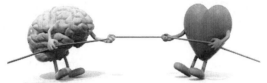

THE EGO **VERSUS**	THE SOUL
False Self	True Self
Me	We
Sadness	Joy
Separation	Unity
Hostility	Friendliness
Blame	Understanding
Pride	Love
Resentment	Forgiveness
Competition	Cooperation
Complain	Gratefulness
Power	Humbleness
Anger	Happiness
Materialism	Spiritualism
Insanity	Wisdom
War	Peace
Cold Hearted	Sympathetic
Intolerance	Tolerance
Service to Self	Service to Others
Self Denial	Self Acceptance

EGO and Belief block what is true

Today it is admirable to be skeptical, but always be open, be the observer. If it looks like a duck and walks and quacks like a duck, it might be a duck. God did not give us a manual to life nor an owner's manual. No one else has the right to judge you, if they have not walked in your shoes and don't know the pain you live with. Their judgment is then based on assumption. Your life should not be ruled living in Fear looking over your shoulder, but living from your heart selfless and asking how you may first serve yourself to become strong so that you may better assist and be of service to others. Mistakes are not bad. God knows that some people are slower learners than others. I am not an authority on the subject but these are my thoughts today. Who knows what thoughts tomorrow will bring as I evolve? Be open to evolve.

Living in your mind leads you to fear that stops you from evolving by suppression. Not minding your business unless it is helping others is a bad habit and can lead to the suspicion and hatred of others who you don't know and may have a lesson for you. Suspicion that someone is going to get you or assuming people are criminals before you have learned something from them is criminal. It is unhealthy and leads you to being acidic and miserable. You miss out so much on what life has to offer from being suspicious of others, living like somehow you are superior because of what you own or where you live or what you drive or what you believe. We are equal. MIRACLES CAN HAPPEN.

The current belief system is the self appointed guardian of the status quo. People are ostracized who step outside the norm which creates an imbalance, and distortion that is unsustainable. Logic and new information of health is rejected in favor of traditional outdated beliefs. Surrendering your power to the current medical system is hurting people. Imagine profound love and your mind will lead you to profound love.

Your mood or frequency is mostly affected by inflammation. Inflammation sucks energy from the body. A healthy body will help you deal with stress, help you to have great relationships and a bright outlook on life and all it has to offer. Disease does not come from the mind, it comes from the body. We live in the 3D body in a 3D world. Thoughts will come more into play as the earth raises in her frequency during the shift into the 5D. Your mind is affected by toxic environments, like a death in the family or a bad marriage, anger, rage, or expectations that are too high. People who have died and have seen "the light" all report a sense of euphoria, so there is nothing to fear about death. But if you live with love in your heart, you can only feel happiness that the newly deceased are in a better place than in one of suffering. RELAX.

Joy is the Compass of Life's Purpose

Try exploring life with an open mind. By applying astrology might help you find your potential. You could go sit by a rushing river if you are a water sign, or you might enjoy sitting in front of a fire if you are a fire sign. If you are an earth sign you could go for a drive to get a view of the valleys from a mountain top. You could learn about what your soul needs if you learn about astrology. Fire and air are the masculine signs that need action and adventure and the earth and water signs are more the loungers of the feminine, which are just ideas that might help you with compatibility as far as relationships go. Chinese astrology can help you with compatibility on probability of long term success. You could learn about yourself through numerology, palmistry or tarot, perhaps an idea put forth you never thought of by reaching into your potential from these type of consultations might help you to let go of limited thinking from the past and ideas for the future you never thought of. This is not for everybody but can help expand your potential using imagination from someone gifted to brainstorm for ideas you never thought of. People refer to lessons as mistakes, but mistakes are negative ways of looking at things. Let's hope you are not in the lesson line up too much! Nothing ventured nothing gained? LISTEN.

Authority can take anything it wants from you if you are in fear. Honey bees are an example where a little smoke is blown into the nest to create fear, and you can then reach into the nest and help yourself.

When you become healthy absent of Fear and Ego you can become the motivator of others?

Motivational speakers and physiotherapists can be cheerleaders until they are blue in the face but if your biology is unhealthy, you will go back to your backache and unfulfilled life when you go home. So your priority is to get your blood healthy first before you seek that kind of counseling.

The most amazing thing that made my jaw hit the floor is that when I offered meal replacement with high density nutrients to people, they thought there might be risks! Ingredients that are life sustaining for your body, but to suggest that they could be at risk? I think to myself, they are in fear. These are irrational thoughts from the same people drinking a coffee and eating a donut, smoking a cigarette who are asking. Eat more nutrients and less toxins is not a profound idea! I found the older the patient, the stronger their belief of the present health care system, and the sicker the patient even stronger their belief. People will die for their beliefs.

Morality is doing what's right regardless of what you're told. Obedience is doing what is told regardless of what is right.

Sleep

Everyone was looking for instant gratification, some sign of confirmation. For instant gratification I guided all of them to a crystal healer who would align their chakras and bring in potential and release negative energy which gave them instant gratification resulting in a boost of energy. This feeling of wellness helped them to move on and try nutrition and detoxing, as the next step which takes longer to feel benefits. For me, the 1 hour crystal healing session made me go home and sleep for 2 days without physical contact from the practitioner. Sleep is the ultimate goal of healing, by releasing spasm to allow you to sleep. It is during sleep that the body repairs itself.

Sleep is critical for cellular recovery. It is the best form of healing that there is. Low magnesium, potassium and vitamin D contribute to poor sleep. Melatonin is a natural source sleep aid that falls off as you age that you can buy cheaply from a health food store. 3mg/5mg tablets you can dissolve under your tongue. Autoimmune kills the alpha Melanocyte Stimulating Hormone that interferes with ability to sleep profoundly and creates depression in patients with that disease. Fractal science describes spasm as stored energy in the body as death that can be expressed mathematically, and energy that flows through you as fractal energy the essence of life. I allow negative energy to flow through me so as to avoid storing energy as spasm in my muscles. Think of it as, "not my energy, it's someone else's" and consciously allow it to go through and release it. Most rage that you see that is unjustified I think of the enraged, is as if they are looking at themselves in their own mirror. They are not mad of what you did, they are just mad period. See them as your child in diapers who needs to be put down for a nap. REST.

Polarity Consciousness = Ego and only cares about self

Massage To remove spasm you press on a tight knot or muscle as hard as you can take, and hold for 30 seconds. The pressure stops the blood flow to the muscle that is in spasm and most of the spasm will dissipate within 30-60 seconds. If the pain or injury is too much to bear because of a damaged muscle, you can do accupressure in the area of sympathetic muscles in the vicinity. But be careful because muscle that is in spasm or pain in the muscle around the injury is protecting the injured muscle. It is how you give instant relief without medication. It is a great benefit to enable sleep which accelerates recovery. If you go to work with that shoulder after releasing the spasm protecting it, you will injure it more than ever if you try to use it normally. Spasm to the body is located principally in 5 points of your body. The most significant spasm held by your body is in your elbows, at the top of your forearm, with palms up. The second point to hit is at the top of your inside shoulder blades where the soft tissue meets. Find the muscle knot and press there for 30 seconds. These 2 points affect your shoulders most. The third point is in the hollow butting up to the hollow under your ears and massaging the bump. These pressure point affects your sleep most. The forth point is in the kidney area on your back, where your stomach muscles meet. The fifth is at the top front of your legs where your legs crease when you bend over. All 5 points affect overall spasm throughout the body, but most of your body's spasm is held in your elbows.

A great way to take out stress, is to sit in the sun as much as possible, best midday because the wavelength of the UVB are the healing rays during that time. It resets your biological clock and the radiant energy penetrates deep into your exposed tissue. This is great for shift workers and people who are exhausted. This is anti-inflammatory and you will lose a few pounds of excess fat during summer through regular sun exposure, without suntan lotion, without burning. It is the non-organic ingredients of suntan lotion and the act of stopping the body converting the sunrays to vitamin D that causes the skin cancer, the sun prevents cancer. There is no better natural way to prevent and eliminate inflammation because it facilitates restful sleep. Stress is best handled from a rested and healthy body. SUNTAN.

If you have the money, massage and acupuncture relieves stress and encourages blood flow. Physio encourages blood flow with electronic equipment. Exercising muscles that are inflamed from autoimmune or from malnourishment should not be encouraged. Chiropractors align your skeletal frame but this should be done after your biology is without inflammation. Inflamed biology of your body is what pulls you out of alignment. I used to go regularly several times a week but found I didn't need the visits once I corrected biology by removing inflammation. Yoga absent of autoimmune was all I needed to cope to feel relaxed and visits to the other practitioners was a luxury and no longer a necessity. You will respond better to treatment when your blood is rich in nutrients and absent of toxins and your cells absent of inflammation.

Mold was the biggest block I found to feeling rested. Sleeping in moldy environments, like in a cool basement, or a room with a broken window seal, or a room with carpet, a leaky roof, a room beside a leaky chimney, you can sleep soundly for 12 hours and wake up and feel exhausted. That is a symptom, a clue that you are in mold. I would tell people to either move or replace the window and remove the source of mold but sleep with the window open and have an extra blanket on to get fresh air to allow you to get restful sleep until you do.

FEAR IS LEARNED

Authority and facts
Freedom from authority makes me happy.

Trust is the most noble attribute a person can have.

Ego will bring you the farthest from spirituality a person can be.

Living in Ego and Fear brings you the farthest away from happiness.

Fear puts limits on potential and aligns you with failure.

If you give up your authority someone will be there to take it from you.

The answer to why is why not?

A sinner is someone who controls another.

It is not about limited motivation, it is more about the cause of limited health.

Chemical companies are taking over the food being served on our dinner plates today.

Sometimes people don't want to hear the truth, lest it destroys their belief.

Your body's ability to heal is greater than anyone has permitted you to believe.

The world will not be destroyed by those who do evil, but by those who watch and do nothing.

Your life is a result of choices. If you don't like your life, review the choices you are making.

The only thing that should work on food is a chef - Scientists are making food an art using poison.

Japan has 54 nuclear reactors built on unstable rock on the unstable convergence of 4 tectonic plates at sea level. Is this planned or are they stupid?

Blood travels about 12000 miles in a day and takes longer if you eat fries and a burger.

Uranium is used in dental porcelain to add whiteness.

Parasites map your body to find weakness.

There is a spike in autism downwind from nuclear plants.

Radiation confuses DNA.

12% drop in SAT university qualification scores for students living down wind of radiation.

The byproduct of Uranium mining is phosphate, sprayed as fertilizer to grow your food.

Anyone who goes to a psychiatrist should have their head read?

Better to live a short life doing what you like, that living a long life doing what you don't like.

What would you do if money was no object?

Change your thoughts to one of self caring and appreciation and life will change.

Spirituality is absent of fear. Try making eye contact with people and smile. Give freely. ALLOW.

People are reduced to that of animal through desperation. Desperation is built into the system.

Solfeggio Frequencies for healing

On Youtube.com that is about an hour long. These healing frequencies you can listen to daily by closing your eyes to relax your mind and release negative thoughts that are of no use to you. Breathe deeply in through your nose.

174 Hertz Is your Foundation

285 Hertz Is for Quantum Cognition

396 Hertz Is for Liberation from Fear

417 Hertz Is for Transmutation

528 Hertz Is for Miracle Meditation and is the love frequency

639 Hertz Is for Integrating Structures

741 Hertz Is for Consciousness Expansion

852 Hertz Is for Awakening.

Consciousness

The desire for truth must be present if you are going to find the answer to health. You need to find success to build on more success. But when you are truly sick, you don't care because you can't. But know that when you are healthy, a pattern of pain needs to be released to raise your vibration, to raise your consciousness. Try to get out of what is "good and bad", and get into your own balance that embraces your needs in the "now", that will be effective and give you power. Other people's rage is their rage and it is not who you are. You are not rage and you let it pass through you with amusement. Don't engage in rage because you don't need it. Rage will not help you thrive. You have to employ willpower to find truth instead of having Authority hand it to you. Compliance only feeds Authority and the "I don't care and herd mentality". This is how you become divorced from consciousness. I don't care if I get mine fuels the system of Control. It is through the mind that Authority controls through a police state society. Snitches are agents of Control. Mind control is where Authority operates. People who have questioned the Authority of Control have been murdered;

John Lennon "Give peace a chance",

Jimmy Hendrix "When the power of love, overcomes the love of power, the world will know peace",

Martin Luther King "I have a dream",

JFK returning the Federal Reserve back to the people got him killed.

Hope is the greatest strength and the greatest weakness of humanity. If you get over fear, you get over weakness. Humanity is in the state they're in because they never understood why. There is only one constant and that is "cause and effect", without it you are powerless. Authority took over health care after WW2 and now is taking over the internet, the highway of information that answers the questions of why.

Light workers are here on earth and need to get healthy now and explain the why to humanity and help them understand and get themselves well. Action for change can only begin when people understand "why".

Actions: Is about your will, using courage, freedom and the exercise of your conscience.
Emotions: Is about your spirit with love, compassion and love.
Thoughts: Is about your mind with intelligence, knowledge and truth.

Losing a significant person in your life raises your risk of having a heart attack the next day by 21 times, and in the following week by 6 times. The risk of heart attacks begins to lower after a month, perhaps as levels of stress hormones begin to decline. People think that the most painful thing in life is losing the one you value, the truth is the most painful thing is losing yourself in the process of valuing someone too much and forgetting that you are special too. Working night shifts negatively affects your health. Women who worked nights had a 40% increased chance of getting breast cancer. Short sleep duration is a public health hazard leading not only to obesity, diabetes and heart disease, but also cancer.

Low vibration frequencies are Judgment, Fear, Resentment, Jealousy, Anger, Rage, Selfishness, Hatred, War, Rage and Arguing live in Ego... fear of the future, fear of the present, fear of the past?

VERSUS

Love, Joy, Happiness, Bliss, Adventure, Passion, Inspiration are high frequencies. People with positive frequency question authority, refuse to draw conclusions from authority. Positive people don't generally judge. Positive people become positive by practicing positive affirmations. Find the good in people, the good in situations, the good in everything and all things.

Watch your life change when you tell someone everyday that they are beautiful.

Everyone says that love hurts, but that is not true...

Loneliness hurts. Rejection hurts, losing someone hurts.

Everyone gets these things confused with love.

Love is the only thing that covers up all pain and makes someone feel wonderful again.

Is there something that frustrates you?

Don't focus on the frustration, but rather on the opportunity for improvement.

Is there something that makes you angry? Instead of being consumed with anger, consider the opportunities for understanding.

Is there something that frightens you? Don't focus on the fear, but rather on the opportunity to better prepare your self.

Is there something that makes you sad? Rather than focusing on the sadness, be thankful for the fact that you care so much.

Is there something that makes you anxious? Don't focus on the anxiety, but rather on the positive purpose you wish to achieve.

No matter what happens, you are always free to choose where to focus.

Choose to focus on the positive, and you'll be choosing great things come to your life.

If you get frustrated or angry, breathe through your nose, frustration will soon dissipate because you can't be in rage if you breathe in through your nose. From a place of calm come your best decisions. Your worst decisions are always made from rage, which doesn't help yourself or anyone. Tune into BNN business news network Canada or CNBC business channel in the US and observe the commentators and guests every second sentence contains the word fear and its bag of synonyms.

Where there is light shone, there is no darkness.

If we are to learn anything about hippies, is that they live in a spirit of high love frequency without control. People that explore their bliss are the happiest of all that walk the earth free from possessions, ego and fear. Listening to the radio, I had to laugh because the radio hosts were making fun of a hippifest. They were making fun of a group of people that were happy and not realizing that hippies are the most evolved people walking the planet. Their footprint is light and they live with love in their hearts and compassion of others at a soul level. These are the people we should be learning from and trying to emulate.

Someone asked me my blood type and I told them, be POSITIVE!

There is a river you must cross but it is occupied by alligators, and you do not have a boat. How do you manage it? Answer next chapter.

Chapter 8

Examples

86% of all Doctor's Visits are Stress Related.

In 1898 Bayer marketed Heroin as a cough medicine for Children.

50% of the US population has chronic illness.

Health care eats up 18% of the US GDP

I believe we could reduce these statistics by over 60% within 60 days.

Alcoholics

It might be helpful if you notice that alcoholic susceptible people without fail, have an extra high sensitivity to their surroundings. For every alcoholic I've talked to is clever, and they admit that the alcohol numbs that sensitivity. It is like having a break to let loose from the constant hyper awareness they experience of their surroundings. It might be helpful for alcoholics if they are aware of this observation to assist them in recovery. The first step is to understanding why. By cleaning your liver and kidneys and taking high density nutrition, together with sunshine and grounding to earth assist to increase the probability of recovery significantly. Just relieving your body of inflammation will give you the euphoria of health. My definition of an alcoholic, is when the alcohol controls you and you don't control it to a point where it doesn't complement your life.

Acne

Is primarily caused by hormones and thought to be by excessive androgen hormones present. The liver filters androgen hormones. Milk is one of those acne aggravators that is rich in hormones that for some by cutting out, reduces acne. UVB midday sunrays is one of the best methods to reduce acne. Sunbeds help too, the kind that have UVB. Beds that use electronic ballasts are safer rather than the magnetic ballasts that interfere with DNA. Using lemons are a method worth investigating.

Allergies and Asthma

I cured my allergies and asthma by cleaning my liver and removing myself from mold. Asthma and allergies can be caused by living in mold even if your liver is clean and functioning properly.

Aloe Vera Gel

Contains over 130 active compounds and 34 amino acids that are beneficial to your skin. You can put it on a burn for amazing relief beyond compare for instant relief. Aloe vera gel is what you want on your skin following any kind of burn. It gives immediate relief from pain and helps to restore the healing of the skin. When a couple ounces is swallowed from a health food store in a glass of water, it has a soothing and almost instant healing effect on everything aloe comes in contact with travelling down your digestive tract. For indigestion and heartburn, there should be nothing better. The dose is a couple of ounces stirred into a cup of water for 3 or 4 days only and perhaps twice a month for maintenance. Try taking it with chlorella, electrolytes, a little apple cider vinegar, and 20 drops of liquid oxygen (not h2o2) from a health food store as a cocktail of healing. If you have Crohn's, cancer or irritation along the digestive tract, it has amazing results that are healing and you might want to consider 10 drops of stabilized oxygen first dose to be sure, before going to 20 drops because of possible reaction to die-off of anaerobic cells for the most sensitive of people.

Alpha Lipoic Acid

Administered by intravenous in a natural path's office is what you take to rebuild your liver on turbo once it is flushed and cleaned. For the urgent you can take it while you are doing a cleanse and flush protocol. ALA is contained in a lot of liver cleanses as an ingredient, and is great for hepatitis disease, along with oxygen to kill the virus (the cause). Alpha lipoic acid lowers blood sugar levels. Its ability to kill free radicals help people with diabetic peripheral neuropathy, who have pain, burning, itching, tingling, and numbness in arms and legs from nerve damage.

Alzheimer

Is caused by, what else, a nutrient deficiency compounded by a toxic liver. Dr Wallach treated a patient who didn't know the name of his wife to recover to the point where that patient was fishing within 60 days of taking broad spectrum meal replacement of 60 minerals, 16 vitamins, 12 amino acids, 3 EFA's, contained in his Tangeyorange proprietary supplement along with an Osteo Fx product you can buy off the InfoWars.com website. That is a News website that broadcasts the real news going on around the country and the world in Syria. You must avoid GMO's and avoid statins. The myelin sheath is made up of 75% of cholesterol by weight. Statin drugs are meant to reduce cholesterol but also dissolve this sheath that exposes patients to symptoms of Alzheimer's and MS. Autoimmune or exposure to mold can dissolve the myelin sheath too. Olestyr is a superior choice to remove cholesterol and neurotoxins of autoimmune patients and has no interaction with body chemistry. Note: the ash left from burnt wood has most of the essential nutrients in it to spread on your garden for nutrient uptake. The trees pull the nutrients from the soil and after the wood is burnt the ashes grow nutrient rich vegetables and fruit in your garden.

Arthritis-pulled muscle

The root cause of back pain is primarily caused by a nutrient deficiency. The trigger is pushing a muscle strenuously when the muscles are tired, overworked and malnourished. There are only two ways arthritis can happen other than trauma. One is either from autoimmune or the other a nutrient deficiency, compromised by a toxic liver. Arthritis and any word that ends with "is", is caused by a nutrient deficiency. If a muscle is called upon to fire to swing a hammer repetitively, that muscle will need nutrition from the blood to feed it. If there are insufficient nutrients in the blood the muscle will be stressed and be put into a state of inflammation. If the muscle continues to be called upon, it will begin to experience pain. If that pain is ignored, there will be permanent damage done by way of scar tissue. Back pain and arthritis are one of the early signals of when disease begins. Robaxacet and muscle relaxants should only be taken before rest or bed when muscle exertion is taking a break.

I've found that Bursitis is one of the "is" that takes longer for cellular repair. Arthritis takes about 10 days to remedy with high density nutrition of broad spectrum meal replacement shakes full of protein, minerals and supplements on a double dose works best along with juicing organic vegetables. Each serving of meal replacement has approximately 10 meals of nutrition stirred into a glass of clean water. It takes about 10 days for cellular absorption to occur.

Pulled muscles, tendonitis, tennis elbow usually happen when the body is malnourished, fatigued, dehydrated and mentally under stress and perhaps where you are absent minded. Arthritis does not happen in your hands. That is called rheumatoid arthritis which is a symptom of autoimmune and is not arthritis. You might find this in your hands, your feet and knees. Inflammation source is from neurotoxins and not so much from nutrient deficiency. Hip replacement is definitely suspected by a nutrient deficiency and occasionally by neurotoxins in the blood from exposure to toxic mold. Muscles fired in an environment where neurotoxins from mold are present will put your muscles into inflammation and it can be nasty. Nice warm dry weather and sunshine or removing yourself from where you live might also get you favorable results. Bad posture is not the answer to your problems. If you don't believe me do the juicing and meal replacements 2x/day for 2 weeks. Yoga is bad posture and removes stored energy from muscles that need to be opened up for nourished blood flow to heal while allowing the negative energy of stress to be released all the while strengthening muscles at the same time.

Anti-Bacterial Soap and sprays

Whatever goes on your hands and gets rubbed in, goes into your fat cells and migrates into the blood stream. Anti-bacterial soap is made up of antibiotics and that substance is going to kill good bacteria in your gut which interferes with nutrient absorption, contributes to obesity, IBS, candida and compromises the immune system and, contributes to depression and drains energy from inflammation. Alcohol or a liquid with oxygen would be a superior substitute. The anti-bacterial soaps are nothing more than antibiotics in disguise. The antibiotic is dispensed at convenient wall stations everywhere now. Triclosan is the active ingredient used in soaps, mouthwash, toothpaste, and toys. Triclosan is a chemical that lowers testosterone and sperm levels in males and triggers early puberty in females. The chemical also contributes to weak hearts and skeletal muscles. Good to know our hospitals and FDA are hard at work?

Antioxidants do an amazing job for eliminating age spots, large freckles, inflammation, disease and cancer. It works subtly to reduce aging by removing free radicals from the body. Glutathione is the most powerful anti-oxidant I know of. The brand I use is not commercially available in volume. You want to take this regularly and especially when you have inflammation and by IV at a natural path's office if you have cancer. It only helps with the burden of disease and is not as powerful as oxygen.

Aspartame and artificial sweetners are now in 6000 consumer products for you to consume. It is the excrement of Ecoli bacteria, and is a cytotoxin that eats your brain cells and later turns to a poisonous form of wood alcohol and eventually to embalming fluid (formaldehyde). It causes obesity by loading up your liver with poison, lowers your IQ, your pH, your immune system and is addictive. Aspartame is by far the most poisonous ingredient sold in a grocery store, but GMO's have recently taken over that honor. Youtube.com "Sweet Misery".

Artificial Flavor

Aborted fetuses are being used in the manufacture of natural flavors. Human aborted fetal cells are being used to develop savory sweet and salt flavor as an ingredient by a Biotech company in Florida. The fetal cells are also being introduced into vaccines. On an episode of the Doctors on TV, they reported that "natural" raspberry flavor is made from the anal sacs of beavers. A quick inquiry confirmed this information as true. You could write a book on this subject and call it, "What I learned at the zoo today".

Artificial Lighting

Is a carcinogen that negatively affects the pineal gland. Eye problems are helped by selenium, zinc, vitamin C, and Axstimanin. Wide spectrum lighting which simulates light closer to outdoor is more calming. Kids with autism are actually suffering from an overload of toxins and heavy metal and therefore have a lower threshold to ambient toxins in their lives. A partial remedy is to not wear sunglasses as much as you possibly can. The sun has healing rays from ambient light that can take spasm out of eye muscles and reset normal biorhythms.

Autism rates have gone up from 1 in 100,000 before the introduction of vaccinations and chemicals in the food chain to 1 in 50 today. Autism is caused by toxic burden and heavy metal overload, and there is a lower threshold to an increasing amount of ambient toxins in their lives as a consequence of drastic increases. That is like 2 trains colliding. I believe that the autism rate of anyone who takes a vaccination is 100%. When a toxic metal called aluminum is added to vaccinations, it intensifies the toxicity of the mercury contained called thimerasol 1000's of times. With the aluminum present, this allows for the mercury to cross the blood brain barrier to start dissolving the brain in areas where the mercury comes in contact. Mercury is the most toxic substance known to man. Children get administered 50,000 parts of mercury by the time they are 6 years old. One part is considered toxic. Aluminum also intensifies the damaging effects of exposure to microwave radiation of wifi, portable phones, cell phones, smart meters, TV's, and video games on brain waves and by its conductive nature, your entire body becomes like an antenna. Also added in the vaccination is squalene to round out the autism cocktail, and the damage is permanent. Squalene is an autoimmune causing adjuvant used to intensify effects of the vaccine, and the results are juvenile rheumatoid arthritis in children. Vaccinations have been proven on 19,000 children to increase the likelihood of being sick 400% on average by a study recently completed by ethical science. Vaccinations are obsolete because of Oxygen therapy using hydrogen peroxide food grade from a health food store, for 1$ taken orally can kill anything that a vaccination is meant for.

PCA is a product of interest because of its success, made by Maxam Nutraceutics out of Oregon to reduce or even eliminate autism. It is a chelation method that binds first with heavy metals found especially in vaccinations for excretion out of the body. You can actually spray it under the tongue. While chelation is commonly administered intravenously using the drug agents dimercaptosuccine acid (DMSA) and dimercaptopropane sulfonate (DMPS), for heavy metal removal, PCA binds with heavy metals first, which makes its effect potent. Patients who switched from chelation to PCA-Rx for treating the autistic victims of vaccinations were extremely pleased with PCA-Rx. Tremendous cognitive gains happen slowly at first and then dramatically. Also taking coconut oil, colloidal silver, chlorella, EFA's daily help with autism mildly. Heavy metal chelation IV is performed by natural paths to eliminate heavy metals. Chlorella and spirulina help with chelation of heavy metals because it crosses the blood brain barrier to bind for elimination as well as being nutritious single celled source super food.

Back and Muscle Pain

Back pain and muscle pain are mostly a form of malnutrition similar to arthritis. Muscles need to be rested and nourished and blood circulating "absent" of neurotoxins from mold. Nutrient deficiency is the major cause combined with a minor cause of a toxic liver. Resting the muscle is best, and infusing with meal replacement for 14 days for repair. Heat and treatment that encourages blood flow repairs quicker if the blood is properly nourished absent of neurotoxins. It is the nutrients in the blood that do the repair work, nothing else can repair an inflamed or pulled muscle, so it would be best to ramp up your meal replacement and watch how it repairs a muscle pain 2-3x faster and for some perhaps 10x faster if you were to take a full glass of meal replacement stirred into water 2-3x per day. You don't want to exercise it until the pain is gone because you will cause permanent damage and scarring and make it prone to more likelihood of reinjuring. I knew people where pain in a muscle like tendonitis could persist for 6 months, and someone taking meal replacement and by juicing organic vegetables, the muscle would be repaired reliably within 2 weeks. Tendonitis or anything ending with "is" is caused by nutrient deficiency compounded by a toxic liver and the trigger is a fatigued muscle. Most skiing accidents happen at the end of the day on the ski hill relying on fatigue muscles. Robax should only be taken when you are ready for rest or sleep. By taking this OTC medication to relax your muscles, you are opening yourself up to more damage if you take it during the day when you are stressing the damaged muscle.

You may take away the pain by physically pressing on the muscle that is in spasm for a minute as hard as you can take and roll it around to fan out the area for 5 to 10 minutes to starve the blood to the muscle. Once the muscle is starved of nutrients, it will let go. A spasmed muscle is the body's natural way to protect a muscle while it repairs but the pain can interfere with sleep, which can lead to other health problems. Be sure to immobilize it after using this technique to remove pain, or you can do even more damage. With back ache, it could be inflamed kidneys possible if it is on both sides just above the hip bones, in which case you want to drink parsley tea.

Bacon

Has a chemical in it that is effective in creating male infertility. Sodium nitrate creates sterility in males. Nitrosamines are created when nitrites are heated. Nitrosamines are a known carcinogen and are intensified, the more you cook bacon.

Bananas

When you get your bananas home, pull them apart and they will sit on your counter longer without over ripening. They are a good source of potassium and mix well in blended fruit smoothies.

Bees

Started dying in droves just after GMO corn was planted, a red flag since corn seeds are treated with neonicotinoid pesticides, which are known to kill insects by attacking their nervous systems. The death of bees really ramped up shortly after Monsanto started buying up Bee Research Labs around the world. Some governments are finally taking action against these toxic chemicals, but not fast enough. For those who aren't aware, there are about 100 crop species that provide 90 percent of food globally and of these, 71 are pollinated by bees. In the US alone, a full one-third of the food supply depends on pollination from bees. If bee colonies continue to be devastated, major food shortages will inevitably result. 25,000 bumblebees were found dead in an Oregon parking lot after 55 trees in the area had been sprayed with Safari, a neonicotinoid insecticide. These chemicals are applied to seeds before planting, allowing the pesticide to be taken up through the plant's vascular system as it grows. As a result, the chemical is expressed in the pollen and nectar of the plant. This is devastating to bees and other pollinating insects. Neonicotinoid pesticides are widely used in large-scale agriculture. They're sold in garden centers, including big-name stores like Home Depot, Lowe's and are even found in seeds and plants you may purchase from your local nurseries. The products that contain poisons are priced similar to food and household products found in the isles of non-organic grocery stores. They are offered at the cheapest price wholesale for wide spread distribution for the bargain hunters for wide spread adoption across the continent by consumers.

Bee Sting

The best I found to remove the swelling and pain was Portland cement. Make a little paste of the powder in your palm with a little water. Then put the wet paste on the sting and expose to the sun which is best or use a hair dryer on low and as it dries it pulls the poison out. It was amazing. Mud could be used in the wilderness as a substitute but it doesn't work as well. If you are allergic to bee stings, carry Portland cement in a small empty pill container in your glove box of your car and your saliva can work to activate it into a paste for relief. As soon as the Portland paste dried, the pain was gone and there was no evidence of there being ever a sting in 2 minutes. Don't hesitate to repeat a few times, it can be amazing.

Brain

The brain burns through oxygen and nutrition to function. Stabilized oxygen (11% ozone) and a meal replacement or juicing vegetables before an exam will raise your IQ. Niacin B3 is thought to help Schizophrenia, mental anxiety, skin rash, and autism. You should substitute coconut oil in place of margarine or butter and get on the road to thriving. It is good for the brain, skin and health. Coconut oil doesn't break down when heated on the stove. Toxins in your food and drink and lack of nutrients, along with low hormones and poor gut flora are the primary source of brain disorders. Inflammation is the main culprit of dementia. Detoxing, chelation and good gut flora with probiotics should be the main focus for brain health.

Breast Cancer

Studies have proven that 83% of breast cancer and cystic breast disease is caused by low iodine. Iodine has been removed in produce grown where the soil has been killed by pesticides. Iodine in salt is woefully inadequate to do anything but prevent goiters, sometimes. Salt is poison that tastes like salt, so throw it in the garbage. Organic Himalayan sea salt is best. Non-organic sea salt is allowed to be mislabeled and contain regular salt. You can buy iodine at a health food store and should be taken as a triple dose for 6 months and re-evaluate (see iodine). The other 17% of breast cancer is caused by xenoestrogens contained in plastics and non-organic underarm deodorant and laundry detergent, the contents of which leave a powerful estrogen film on the sheets you sleep in and the clothes you wear to be absorbed into the bloodstream through the skin.

Building Codes

Were out of line in the past and still are. Lead pipes were used in the past as an element to transport our drinking water. Lead is highly toxic and creates brain disorders and makes you vomit. Aluminum wiring was used in houses widespread in the 70's. Any electrician who evaluated it would throw it to the curb in 60 seconds after trying to bend or use it. Cost was the reason for adoption and it was responsible for numerous fires because of aluminum's low retentivity. When the screw is pressed down on the wire in the switch or plug device the wire collapses under the pressure like liquid over time and a gap in current flow to the device, causes it to spark, overheat and fires ensued. Aluminum wire was approved or was mandated by a safety authority. No safety authority in their right mind would approve aluminum wiring in homes.

Asbestos, who did the science on that product? It caused a lot of respiratory illness and deaths and is before the courts and clean up of this product out of buildings is extensive.

Today, I see problems with building codes for example, with heat registers near windows. This practice reduces efficiency of buildings by perhaps 20%. The heat loss at a cold window 32F/0C in the winter is inefficient when it meets hot air coming directly from a vent 120F/50C. If the heat from the vent had a chance to merge with the ambient air of the room, at 72F/22C before coming in contact with the 32F/0C at the window, the heat loss would be much less. The energy differential would be only 40F/22C instead of 90F/50C. To prove my point, use a thermal imaging gun to show the picture of heat loss while the furnace is on in your building. It will look like it is on fire.

Another lame-brain building code places people to live in plastic bags called vapor barriers in climates across North America where temperatures are up and down by as much as 100F/38C. It is mandatory in modern homes built since the 70's and has caused havoc in the community with autoimmune. If we could get statistics of autoimmune disease on a timely basis, you would see a disaster with this particular building code. All you need is a hole from a picture or mirror to puncture the seal or miss a flap in a corner with tape, and you have a nest of mold that can contaminate a home behind the drywall. Old windows with broken seals drip water behind the vapor barriers commonly, and create toxic air that leads to autoimmune disease, asthma and allergy problems. Particle board and carpet are petri dishes for toxic mold. People living in basements are a recipe for toxic mold exposure, as partition walls are put up and ventilation behind next to cold walls is cut off.

CANCER

Cancer is very easy to understand, easy to get rid of and a symptom of excessive inflammation over a long period of time. The inflammation of cancer is caused by an imbalance in one or more of the 5 elements of the Matrix. Balance the five elements that are deficient or in the case of toxins, "proficient", and burn it out with oxygen, #8 in the periodic table. Cancerous, mutated cells thrive in anaerobic, oxygen-lacking environments. The prime symptom of cancer is the replacement of the respiration of oxygen in normal body cells by a fermentation of sugar in an environment that lacks oxygen. Another symptom of cancer is a dysfunction in the cell's mitochondria that play a major role in cell respiration, which leads to further complications with apoptosis (programmed cell death).

Your body doesn't eliminate cancer because of being alkaline, that is just a symptom of a healthy body that is free of inflammation from cancer. It is cause and effect. There is a lot of misleading information about curing cancer. Curing cancer as with almost any disease is about embracing health, through nutrient loading, elimination and avoidance of toxins, and being absent of autoimmune symptoms with hormones in balance. Embrace health and you leave disease and cancer in the rear view mirror. It is best to wait do hormone replacement until after you are cleared of disease. The best nutrient your body needs is the one you are lowest in, so why not give your body all of them? Go to chapter 2 for the weight loss list of do's and don'ts and chapter 6 for cleansing and this chapter for oxygen. If your body needs EFA's, it will lower cancer symptoms by lowering inflammation by addressing the imbalance, once the deprivation of that substance is satisfied. Omega oils, the air you breathe are nutrients. Cancer is easy to beat, and should be viewed as a nuisance and nothing you should be afraid of. Cancer has always been a rare illness, except in industrialized nations during the past 60 years. Human genes have not significantly changed for thousands of years, but cancer is afflicting nearly half of the population as a cause of death? The evidence is clear with 50% of the population in the US having a chronic disease without any change to genes, proof that the problem is external.

Cancer can also be caused by radiation from exposure to, microwaves, radiation from your cell phone, wifi, portable phones in your home, going through body scans at the airport, truckers going through customs and getting "nuked". CT scans and Galleon scans at the hospital, fallout from nuclear catastrophes like Fukishima and being downwind from nuclear power plants have shown to be serious sources of radiation. One afternoon, I listened to a doctor talking on NaturalNews.com about 400 cures available to treat cancer patients. The cures are available, but underground in North America. H2O2 hydrogen peroxide is the cheapest being $7 at your health food store. I found a dozen cures myself and the few that I tried worked, after 6 rounds of chemo didn't. When my cancer came back with a vengeance, my immunoglobulin A (IGa) was undetectable. That is 75% of my immune system gone and the other 25% compromised, I would have been dead doing chemo over again with an immune system barely functioning. I read that the statistical success rate for cancer is in the mid-single digits (that falsely includes me as a success) to be alive after 5 years and that statistic has barely budged since it came out over 60 years ago. I believe that chemo has a single % success rate above 0% only because people change their lifestyles and diet once they contract cancer. The cures I found had statistical success of over 80%, and the different types of oxygen treatments are closer to 100% success, provided the 5 elements are addressed.

For cancer and severe diseases, you want to do more protocols to embrace health listed in chapter 2, as well you want to do extensive organ cleansing, and getting nutrition to your cells for repair are important. We all need organic juicing, fruits, vegetables and salads, high density protein meal replacement, supplements and avoid toxins like tap water and regular white salt, milk, anything with GMO from flour, cereal, avoid meat from a 4 legged animal, white salt, and anything with sugar. Sugar feeds cancer. Switch to organic everything from food to salt to underarm deodorant!

High Quality supplements that "lower" cancer and disease:

- Vitamin D 10,000-50-000iu/day and get lots of midday sun without burning-no lotion, lowers inflammation. 50,000 tablets should be temporary, of not more than 6 months. Vitamin D doesn't start to work until you take 5,000iu/day.
- High quality tumeric lowers inflammation from a health food store
- EFA's essential fatty acids lowers inflammation
- Krill is a form of an EFA but is more bioavailable to your body but costs more
- Ubiquinol is expensive but improves energy
- B12 is inexpensive and boosts energy too. Some weight loss clinics use it to boost energy of patients as they bring them close to death on a starvation diet.
- Chlorella or spirulina, a teaspoon in a glass of water a day, is both a bioavailable nutrient and detoxifying
- Aloe vera gel 1-2 oz. in a glass of water heals everything it touches down the digestive tract.
- Wheat grass has a lot of nutrients and is live food in an ice cube I would put in my drinks that would help lower inflammation. Given to dogs with their food helps reduce veterinarian bills by up to 90% according to some breeders. Also try trace minerals in the pet dish daily.
- Iodine especially high dose for bone and breast cancer (high cause of these cancers). Low iodine contributes to all cancers and inflammation. Taking Iodine lowers inflammation. There is currently an epidemic in North America of low iodine caused by that nutrition being removed from food, and loss is

accelerated by drinking and bathing in tap water from a municipal system bleaching out your iodine. Low iodine deactivates your metabolism, which causes obesity and inflammation/disease and is worth repeating that it is the most important supplement everyone needs to take!

- Vitamin D ranks as #2 for lowering inflammation.
  Probiotics and digestive enzymes with regular meals for high quality nutrient absorption. All cancer patients have high candida from bad bacteria in their guts. Probiotics should be renamed perhaps "digestive bacteria" or "essential bacteria" similar to essential fatty acids.
- BENTONITE clay (about 15% as effective as Csm for autoimmune) on an empty stomach binds to heavy metals and clearing toxins from inhaling in chemtrails. Bentonite can cause constipation, so perhaps increase fruit intake as a suggestion.

Cancer - antioxidants: that "lower" cancer and inflammation.

Work like that of oxygen taking out diseased and mutated cells by cell apoptosis, and free radicals to help heal cancer. Healthy cells can be more effectively revitalized with nutrition by using anti-oxidants.

- PINE BARK supplement is a powerful antioxidant. Antioxidants deactivate highly destructive free radicals, which are chemicals that damage cells and contribute to many diseases, ranging from stroke and heart attacks to degenerative diseases such as Alzheimer's, and contribute to aging. A lot of mental disorders are inflammation running rampant over time and can be prevented and relieved with nutrition in a body absent of toxins. Scar tissue is permanent, so time is of the essence.
- VITAMIN C high dose of quality. Ascorbic acid does not give you vitamin C useful to your body. Citrus bioflavonoids are useful.
- GLUTATHIONE is 100x stronger than vitamin C. Both are antioxidants and remove unhealthy cells from the body by cell apoptosis. It also helps remove toxins and helps with cellular absorption.

- VITAMIN E, Selenium, and Zinc are examples of subtle antioxidants.
- AMBROTOSE by Mannatech Inc, for cancer and reducing inflammation. I read that it works well in cellular communication, which is what an antioxidant does. It determines if a cell is healthy and restores it with nourishment or eliminates it. I heard from a doctor back in 2000, that the architecture of the molecule has the added benefit that it punctures cancer cells dead on contact. It is effective in the treatment of Lupus, MS and Chronic Fatigue symptoms but does not get rid of the cause which is mold and the removal of neurotoxins. Mannatech has great products worth trying, and has been hounded by the FDA for years, so you know the company must be good! FDA seems to act to protect drug patents and not in the interests of patient care.

"Subtle" ways to get rid of cancer and inflammation:

- B17 or LAETRILE from organic apricot seeds (take 1 every hour unless you have diverticulitis) kills cancer cells on contact. B17 or otherwise known as laetrile worked very well for me and others. You can eat one organic apricot seed an hour while you are awake or can bring it in from Mexico in tablet form. The molecule of the vitamin is tightly bound around cynanide. When Laetrile comes in contact with a cancer cell it releases the cyanide into the cancer cell, killing it. It is an example of mother-nature working perfectly and is a great supplement to prevent cancer. Another name for laetrile is nitrilocides which are abundant in blueberries. Laetrile works well with Larch tree extract to lower TNF-b1 to make it more effective.
- FLOR-ESSENCE is something I took that is similar to Essiac but has 4 more ingredients to help fight cancer. It is a nutritional liquid sold in a bottle brought to market and rejected by the FDA. Rene Caisse, a Canadian nurse from Bracebridge Canada, who claimed that it had been given to her by a patient and that the recipe was derived from an Ontario Ojibwa medicine man. The name "Essiac" is Caisse's surname spelled backwards.

- LARCH TREE EXTRACT contains arabinogalactans that effectively lowers TNF-bl.

   Larch Extract by Source Naturals CA., has been shown to decrease NF-kappaB, and TNF-bland works by "cleaning up" the lymphatic system. It reduces pain in Auto Immune patients and helps your body's immune system to fight cancer, by enabling cell apoptosis (death of diseased cells) of your own body's immune system. Cancer cells have a tough protein covering and with TNF-bl lowered, the body can then join in the fight against cancer. With TNF high the enzyme coating on the cancer cell, will not allow the body's immune system to penetrate it.

Profound ways to "eliminate" cancer.

- H2O2 HRYDROGEN PEROXIDE food grade, they used hydrogen peroxide on the battle field during WWI, to get rid of pneumonia in a day or two. It is also used to get rid of cancer within a month, at full dose. Note: Oxygen only works on symptoms of inflammation and not the cause of cancer. Cancer is a symptom of inflammation and autoimmune is a symptom of neurotoxins. Oxygen would work on Lyme disease to kill the spirochete bacteria but be careful of Herxheimer's reaction from overwhelming toxic die-off of organisms and candida, so be cautious. The only exception oxygen is unlikely to resolve, is cancer sourced from radiation. The h2o2 can bring back normal cells and lungs to pink for pennies a day in patients with COPD and emphysema too, as long as scar tissue is not too severe. For h2o2 food grade used externally, about ½ cup (4oz) in the bathtub is great for soaking in. It helps to reduce toxic burden from the outside externally. Use a liter/quart a week in your hot tub instead of chemicals you currently use. The chemicals cause dozens of diseases. There are different ways to get oxygen into the body. One is cardio activity that prevents disease, another is hyperbaric chamber and another is hydrogen peroxide food grade administered by a natural path by IV.
- OZONE is another method of getting oxygen into your body. Ozone by "IV" therapy takes out AIDS and cancer and you can

get in Mexico, and some underground clinics in the US that are off the radar map of the FDA.

- MMS is an effective product that the government is actively trying to get out of your country, because it works so well at targeting anaerobic cells (cancer and disease). It is chlorine dioxide and is very potent. 2nd cheapest on the list of various oxygen delivery methods to the cells.

- HYPERBARIC CHAMBER is mid-priced and works the least effective at getting oxygen into your cells under pressure to lower inflammation.

- VITAMIN C an antioxidant, 100cc 3x/week by IV works very fast at eliminating cancer.

- BLACK SALVE was used extensively before allopathic medicine started to take over in the 1920's, when it was banned.

- ROYAL RIFE in the 1920's developed a microscope that could magnify diseased cells at 60,000x power and he observed them die when he applied a frequency to that organism under his microscope matching its resonant frequency from an external power source. He could apply a specific frequency, specific to a diseased cell's harmonic frequency and observe it explode. So using the resonant frequency of that cell of the particular disease, could be taken out of the patient by holding onto 2 electrical probe conductors wired back to his frequency generating machine for an hour of 6-10 sessions. Rife is still used today and can take out cancer or candida from a patient. His method could work for any disease or parasite that didn't belong in your body. His equipment, notes and assets were seized and Rife was arrested with guns pointed at his head. His brilliant work and equipment was confiscated and his equipment has never been duplicated because all current equipment used today is missing the feed-back loop that connects back to the patient.

- Dr. HULDA CLARK who practiced with some radical cleanses some from the Egyptian years also incorporated Rife technology in her natural path clinic. It was when she practicing cleanses of the kidneys and liver and gallbladder that made surgery on those organs virtually obsolete, that she was forced to leave the US, to practice down in Mexico using Rife technology to take out disease cells and along with her cleanse protocols. She specialized in preventing and curing disease focused on healing the liver. She just passed away but her book and her formula can be bought at Clarkia.com, used to kill parasites in the liver.

- Dr. HARRY HOXSEY was a successful story of a doctor that observed his horse dying of cancer. He put the horse out to pasture for her last days and observed her eating unusual flowers and grasses in the field she didn't normally eat. For weeks he followed the horse and made a record of what she ate and watched the horse recover from cancer. From the record of what she ate, Dr. Hoxsey made a mixture of the same ingredients, wondering if the herbal mixture would work on humans. He applied it topically and patients ingested the formula as well. The formula worked and the treatment was cheap. The success rate was over 80% which is more than 10x more effective than chemo from what is statistically reported. He offered the cure cheaply but had his 50 or so clinics shut down and he was chased to Mexico to continue his practice there.

- Dr. BURZYNSKI in Houston Texas came up with a method to cure cancer that has a high success rate, after looking at his impressive statistics. Antineoplastons are peptides and derivatives of amino acids that act as genetic switches. They turn off the oncogenes that cause cancer, and turn on or activate tumor suppressor genes that fight cancer. His success rate is also over 80% with statistics including patients the cancer wards have given up on. He had the FDA raid his place with guns and he was facing 300 years in jail and $400 million in fines for saving people's lives. They came at him trial after trial for over a decade. He was acquitted at every trial and continues to practice from his clinic in Houston, Texas. The FDA was forced to give him a sliver of concession by allowing him to do clinical treatment for brain cancers, but his cure works for all parts of the body. He has a good heart and he has been violated to the point where I question the usefulness of the FDA. His story can be found on You Tube.

- Dr. GERSON cured cancer by using a method of juicing vegetables and coffee enemas. He too got chased out of the country with his successful idea. His juicer is a slick on-the-counter 2 ton press and along with coffee enemas to gently remove toxins he had success. His method is another example of nutrition and cleansing to reduce inflammation to allow your own body to cure disease itself. His juicer is priced at 2500$ and delivers the best nutrients available from a juicer.

- MARIJUANA juicing is another effective method to reduce cancer. It is 65x more effective juiced than smoking it. The ban on marijuana is thought to have happened because hemp made a better paper (without environmental damage) than using pulp paper. Also hemp was a superior material to cotton for clothing and could cure cancer. It's another example of conflict of interest, restricting true capitalism.

- OVER 400 CURES I tuned in to a radio broadcast on the internet presented by Mike Adams of NaturalNews.com for an afternoon and listened to a US trained board certified doctor talk about over 400 cures and methods to cure cancer available today... here...now and some cheap. A session of 6 chemo treatments costs a 100 thousand dollars plus the cost of recovery. Why are they called treatments? They should be called torture sessions. The 400+ treatment methods are a fraction of the cost and you don't have to miss work! Every cancer patient needs to cleanse and use high density nutrients to lower inflammation. Some supplements are essential, and hormones should be rebalanced at the end of the disease and not during. The cancer rate is 7x more likely than of those who drink Fluoride in their drinking water.

End of Cancer.

Cannibis

34 studies now confirm that cannibis can be used to rid the body of cancer and is 65x stronger juiced than smoked. It was banned for corporate agendas and not for the good of the community. The cannabinoid compounds naturally found in many varieties of cannabis, help children with autism disorders experience dramatic behavioral improvements, and it is found naturally occurring in breast milk.

Cardio

Oxygen is a nutrient. Daily exercise increases your capacity of your capillaries to exchange oxygen. Increased oxygen eliminates toxic anaerobic cells and there is an added benefit of sweating, in that it eliminates toxins, provided you replace with toxic free water. Movement of your body squeezes toxins from your cells and body parts, and exercise increases endorphins, a mood elevator. It's best to exercise 12-30 minutes in the morning to speed up metabolism throughout the day and follow with a meal replacement stirred into a glass of water.

Cat Food

Cats are carnivores (meat eaters) suited for protein and fat. Dry dental diets are not effective, they need nutrients found in animal protein to survive. Cats lack the amylase enzymes for carbohydrate digestion. Dry cat kibble has carbohydrates as the first ingredient. Best to buy dog and cat food at a health food store. Putting a pinch of wheat grass in the dish of your animals helps to reduce vet bills.

Compact fluorescent light bulbs (CFL)

The efficient bulbs contain mercury powder/vapor and burn with high energy dangerous ultra-violet light. When a bulb breaks you should ventilate the home and avoid skin contact. The small bulbs typically have tubes that curl that emit light.

Charities

A yearlong investigation to evaluate America's charities was done. Investigators found that on average, charities contribute less than four cents of cash collected to aid their cause for every dollar they collect. Many nonprofits are less charitable than for-profits, paying six-figure salaries to their CEOs while contributing relatively nothing to their supposed cause. There is a false sense assumed by the population that everything is being done to help the sick, diseased, impoverished, and the young. Below is a highlight of how wrong people's assumptions are by a Florida newspaper and CNN.

- Kids Wish Network spent only 2.5% on direct cash aid of $127.8 million raised.

- Cancer fund of America spent 0.9% of total funds raised of $98 million.
- Breast Cancer Relief Foundation spent 2.2% to help the cause.
- International Union of Police Associations spent just 0.5% on their cause.

I think the charity we need to give to is Farm Aid supported by Willie Nelson and their initiatives to get rid of GMO's and declare Monsanto a criminal organization. We need our farmers healthy so we can keep what food we can healthy. Perhaps it is our honest farmers we can recruit to lead our countries as politicians and to lead the attack against Monsanto. Those are the doors that need to be shut and assets seized.

Give to "MoveOn.org" to get rid of GMO's.
Give to "OrganicConsumers.org" to stop war and for humanitarian causes.
Avaaz@avaaz.Org appear to be doing good work to stop war and Monsanto.

Chelation Therapy

Is used as a treatment for acute mercury, iron, arsenic, lead, uranium, plutonium and other forms of toxic metal poisoning. The chelating agent may be administered intravenously, intramuscularly, or orally, depending on the agent and the type of poisoning. Natural path doctors are the popular administrators of this therapy and are most knowledgeable.

ALA - is used for the acceleration in rebuilding of damaged livers. Great for Hepatitis victims and because Hepatitis is caused by a virus, Oxygen therapy should be considered to get rid of the cause of the problem, the virus. Great for diabetes patients, administered by a natural path.

BAL - Dimercaprol used in Britain to remove arsenic, mercury, lead poisoning.

DMPS - is used for acute mercury and arsenic poison removal.

DMSA - is used for mercury from contamination of dental fillings, lead and arsenic poison removal as well.

Deferoxamine - for iron poisoning.

EDTA - is best for lead poison removal.

Penicillamine - for copper, gold, arsenic, lead poisoning.

Chemicals vs Bacteria

More and more the health care system is having us ignore the problem of chemicals in our food and environment and has us focusing more on bacteria. Bacteria is not a problem, the problem is the overwhelming toxins in our bodies. Your body functioning without chemicals strengthens your body's immune system by raising your pH. The real problem emerging is the presence of chemicals compromising the immune system that makes you more susceptible to bacteria and we are left with the "treat the symptom" solution of vaccinations, more antibiotics and more visits to the doctor more than ever. The presence of mold in buildings and the engineering behind the building code itself has destroyed a significant percentage of the population's immunity. I can see the compromised immunity engineered on several levels. The problem are the chemicals in our blood and cells wreaking havoc. The only solution is to eliminate chemicals and poison from our water, food and air and move back to our origins or organic nutrition absent of toxins.

IMMATURE IS A WORD BORING PEOPLE USE TO DESCRIBE FUN PEOPLE.

Chemo

Something as strong as chemo that doesn't work the first time, you might not want to do a second time. Each course requires usually 6 rounds and that permanently damages your kidneys, liver, brain, and knocks out 75% of your immune system. IGa becomes undetectable by a blood test and damages the other 25%. Most people die of pneumonia and cancer patients have almost no immune system when cancer returns. When you take chemo, most don't die from cancer, you usually die from damage to your organs compounded by immune system deficiencies. It is poison derived from the technologies of agent orange, a group of companies taking over agriculture and poison on your dinner plate. Chemo brings your whole body close to death, which is the opposite direction to what I found was necessary to thrive, and contrary to common sense. Inflammation and subsequent disease is the absence of health.

Chlorella and Spirulina

Are green chlorophyll super foods from fresh water algae that is rich in protein and can help boost your immune system and regulate cholesterol and blood as well are essential for fighting disease. Both are a natural heavy metal detoxifier and good for detoxifying and protecting the liver. Chlorella is 68% complete protein and contains rich stores of antioxidants, essential fatty acids, vitamins, minerals and both are good for the autistic who have heavy metal toxicity from vaccinations because it is able to cross the blood brain barrier to have positive affects to bind and help flush out heavy metals. Nutrient loading and the subtle benefits can be seen within a couple of weeks of daily consumption of a teaspoon in a glass of water or juice.

Cholesterol

Cholesterol is good for you. It is an essential protein for the building blocks of cellular life. Cholesterol is primarily caused by eating HFCS, high fructose corn syrup and it is in just about everything in a grocery store. It is a refined protein that is a poison that tastes like sugar. HFCS and sugar act like sandpaper on your veins and arteries creating inflammation. The scab material for healing the inflammation is a protein called cholesterol. Bad cholesterol and bad cholesterol ratios are caused by poor diet, rich in sweets and sugars of low bioavailability of food your body doesn't recognize. Problems arise when a toxic liver loses its ability to eliminate excess cholesterol while a large inflow continues with poor diet. I think statin drugs were brought out to replace Olestyr to remove cholesterol, which was curing autoimmune patients and raising too many questions. Olestyr is superior to remove cholesterol in that it has no interaction with the chemistry of your body, it only passes through. People who have bad gut flora ratios have trouble passing this substance and it can cause constipation which can be managed with the IBS protocol of oxygen and probiotics. Cholesterol should be gone after 30 days of organic shopping, meal replacement for protein and minerals, along with organic fruit, vegetables and juicing, flushing and cleaning the liver. It's also about lowering inflammation so take EFA's but better is Krill which is the most bio-available. Omega 3 oils and Krill favorably change the balance of good (HDL) cholesterol to bad (LDL) cholesterol. LDL and HDL's are proteins that transport cholesterol. 87% of a cell comes from cholesterol, so lowering cholesterol is bad for you. But cholesterol is good for you, so you want to desperately get rid of statins. It is estimated that maybe 1% of the population needs to have their "absolute" cholesterol lowered. If you can adopt the Do's/Don'ts list in Chapter 2, it should get you out of the woods. It is cholesterol + protein + hormones + amino acids in a toxic-free environment that are essential for cellular production and muscle growth. Statin drugs will cause an array of other diseases because you lose your body's ability to repair itself. If you take statin medication think about throwing them in the garbage and try taking cholestyramine (Olestyr) instead, especially if you have autoimmune. You will have to insist on it, because it seems that the doctors drag their feet to prescribe it.

I talked to a specialist that said that someone with 3 arteries blocked 80% avoided surgery by consuming a raw food diet in 10 days. An organic raw food diet is food that is alive, having a high life force energy will change the chemistry of your blood. On this diet your body will have a chance to detoxify itself, return to proper gene predisposition, restoring inflamed malnourished cells with spiked nutrients that are bioavailable that your body recognizes. Stroke, heart attack, and heart disease become virtually obsolete. Testosterone is 95% cholesterol by weight, so say good bye to sex life if you take statin drugs that lower cholesterol. B1 or thiamine deficiency is the primary cause of congestive heart failure. Dietary cholesterol in eggs has nothing to do with cholesterol in the blood and organic free range eggs are good for you and actually help lower cholesterol problems.

Cigarettes

The whole time I was growing up, I saw ads that had doctors say that smoking was good for you. Where did that science come from? When I was 8 years old, I concluded that inhaling smoke was bad for you when I saw people being carried out of burning houses by firemen who didn't look well, some like rag dolls. It took the modern world 60 years to realize that inhaling cigarette smoke was dangerous for you? Today posters display the hazards of smoking. On that poster are the various chemicals that are contained in cigarettes. When did these chemicals start getting added? The list chemicals are contained in one cigarette below:

Methoprene a chemical used to get rid of insects,

Benzoprene the most potent cancer causing chemical in the world,

Arsenic a deadly poison similar to the ingredient in your drinking water,

Acetone a nail polish remover,

Lead which stunts growth, damages brain and causes vomiting,

Formaldehyde an embalming fluid that morgues use to preserve dead bodies, it also causes cancer, damages lungs, skin, digestive system, life can't exist it in this chemical,

Turpentine used as a toxic paint stripper,

Butane a key component of gasoline,

Propylene Glycol delivers toxic nicotine to the brain,

Cadmium damages liver, kidneys,

Ammonia adds flavor and helps the body absorb more nicotine,

Benzene causes cancer and is a chemical used to make pesticides, gas and detergent.

Smoking is a source of toxins which harms the liver (#4 on the list of elements), weakens the lungs and interferes with nutrient absorption (#3 on the list of elements) by killing digestive enzymes of the food you eat. Smoking also interferes with your lung's ability to exchange oxygen in the capillaries, which reduces oxygen in your brain and your body, which inhibits its ability to kill anaerobic diseased cells in your body, which leads to cancer. I don't think it is enough to say smoking is bad for you, explaining how brings the meaning to life.

The science about the benefits of smoking didn't make sense to me when I was 8 years old and neither does most of what I hear today about advice our government and official agencies are advising. They said smoking was good for you during WW2 to calm your nerves, then they said smoking won't harm you, then they said more science research is needed, then they said that smoking could harm you, then they said smoking is bad for you, then they said smoking can kill you, then they said that smoking will kill you, then they said you can't smoke cigarettes here and there, then they said you can't smoke cigarettes in your car and just about everywhere? Truth is sold to the highest bidder.

Coffee

Coffee is a diuretic which dehydrates your body. Dehydrating your body can't help but make your body toxic. If you drink a cup of coffee, it takes about 4 cups of water to rehydrate. It also constricts your blood vessels which puts your body into stress, a flight or fight situation. I call coffee heart attack juice. The constricting of blood vessels increases blood pressure, which creates a synthetic alertness that over the long term, is unhealthy. It is an artificial stimulant that can't be matched to the alertness of real health. The boost in present alertness of drinking coffee, comes at a price, by borrowing energy from the future and bringing that energy into the present. If you read about cholesterol, you can read about how cream and sugar are major contributors to bad LDL cholesterol.

If you have to drink coffee it should be drank ½ hour before a meal or 1 hour after. Coffee kills the enzymes and subsequently the bio availability of nutrients to your cells of what you eat with it. This contributes to arthritis and obesity and an increase in cholesterol.

Soda, alcohol, smoking, and microwaves do similar damage to nutrient absorption as coffee does, by killing the digestive enzymes and nutrient absorption that leads to inflammation, weight problems, leading to disease over time. All a source of toxins which lead to the liver becoming further burdened. Coffee shops should switch to juicing vegetables and dispensing this out the window with stabilized oxygen (11% ozone) added. It will wake you up and raise your IQ more than any coffee could ever hope to.

Colds

I think that colds are a symptom of sleep deprivation, energy draining spasm in the body and weakened immune systems. All 3 are related to one another. I've heard a plausible explanation that they can be caused by dying parasites in the liver. To rid yourself of a cold, try exposing your face and body to warm sunlight. If you work shift work, take 20-30 minutes after your shift to sit in the sun, it resets your biological clock and actually relaxes you for restful sleep. Radiant heat sauna, putting your face close to a fire or a radiant heater, massage, a hot shower, hot bath, all work well to remove spasm from the body which allows for restful sleep. With your liver clean and absent of mold and allergies, sneezing is a signaler of a cold coming on. Evaluate whether you have a "nap in you" when you sneeze.

Looking at the sky can entice sneezing, and if that happens, face the heat of the sun to get you ready for that nap you are deprived of. Your body talks to you in mysterious ways. Try oil of oregano capsules or drops for a day or two if you feel a cold coming on. Listen to your body's signals, it talks to you.

Colds because of moldy environments

Colds happen to people in moldy environments because mold reduces your immune system and can profoundly. Air Conditioners and ductwork are awesome carriers of this lurking problem. Did you notice in school it is the same kids that are sick and away at the same time at the arrival of the cold season when furnaces are turned on?

These will be the kids living in the house that had flood damage, a leaky roof or windows, an old house, or they are living in a basement. Mold destroys the immune system that lead to the symptoms of colds and sore throats, recurrent infections, headaches, poor sleep, boils, laziness, lethargy, memory problems, inability to learn and concentrate, gum infections and dental problems. This is for adults as well. Air conditioners in your hotel room might be the root cause of your Montezuma's revenge you might think is food poisoning, headaches, "I partied or drank too much" syndrome while on, or coming back from your vacation. Vacation resorts are bad for air conditioners that don't drain the water from their units and have the influence of warm moist air coming off the ocean to foster colonies of mold. Don't hesitate to sleep with the door or a window open for fresh air while on vacation. You will know the 1st morning, whether you have a problem in your hotel room. The worst rooms will have a musty smell.

Colloidal Silver

Accelerates your healing from a cold and helps boost your immune system. Swished around under the tongue and swallowed helps eliminate heavy metals, kills bacteria and viruses. It works very subtly over time and well with antibiotics. It is a chelator of toxic heavy metals.

Concsiousness

Consciousness is where everything exists and nothing is judged. Oneness just is. Judgement, then is of someone who doesn't understand? Consciousness is the quality or state of being aware of an external object or something within one self. It has been defined as awareness, the ability to experience or to feel, to be awake. "Being" with someone and "sharing" with someone are 2 different things. The body is made up of 4 elements, carbon, oxygen, hydrogen and nitrogen. There is a link between emotion and genetics. Fear has a long wave of emotion and Love has short more frequent waves that interact with DNA more often. The earth's frequency, which affects our body at a cellular level, has been at 7.8hz as a base resonant frequency for 1000's of years. It has been increasing according to the fibonacci sequence since 1986 on its way up to 13.8 hz in the next couple of years. This base frequency of earth is known as the Schumann cavity resonance." Our bodies respond to that electromagnetic pulse. The cells receive their pulse from the brain, which receives its pulse from the heart, which receives its pulse from the earth, which receives its pulse from the solar system, which receives its pulse from the galaxy, which receives its pulse from the universe. We share our pulse with everything in existence as "one." As the earth's frequency increases more of the DNA codes are starting to activate. This is known as ascension. With ascension the human body will vibrate faster in sync with the increasing vibration of the earth. As you start to vibrate faster, toxic food and life habits will start to become more toxic. It is all the more important to embrace health and to shed toxins to experience personal success. Hatred, fear and poor health do not belong in a higher vibration going forward. This is the time to purge toxins, practice yoga and meditation really out of necessity. This is important.

Diabetes

Is about inflammation of the pancreas that leads to problems with leptin-glucose ratios. A bioavailable diet of nutrients your body recognizes absent of toxins helps to control the symptom of inflammation of the organ. The inflammation can be caused many things. Perhaps by exposure to biotoxins, regular alcohol consumption, poor diet and health that turns bile to a sludge that contributes to the formation of gallstones that back up toxins interfering and damaging the pancreas. The pancreas is the power center of the body because it controls blood sugar. High quality diet, along with liver flushes of gallstones and cleanses really help with symptoms and allows time free to reduce inflammation and for natural repair of the organ. Antioxidants like glutathione work well to reduce inflammation. The guide to lose weight in chapter 2 is the same guide to get rid of cholesterol, diabetes, cancer, and just about every disease there is. When the level of one's health falls, the rocks of disease expose themselves. By raising overall health using the 5 elements of the Matrix, those exposed rocks can submerge safely below a raised level of overall health. Health problems you are born with, you will die with. Recovery of the diabetes depends on how damaged the organ is. Taking a Chromium supplement helps diabetes symptoms and so does cutting out wheat. Complex whole wheat and grains raises blood sugar and triggers resistance to insulin, visceral fat more effectively than sugar itself. Wheat is perfect for contributing to obesity, IBS, and lowering the celiac threshold of intolerance for autoimmune patients exposed to mold. Wheat is added to salad dressings, soups, prepared food, frozen food and even licorice. Another reason to avoid non-organic food in regular grocery stores. Alpha lipoic acid lowers blood sugar levels. Its ability to kill free radicals help people with diabetic peripheral neuropathy, who have pain, burning, itching, tingling, and numbness in arms and legs from nerve damage. Diabetes is common amongst autoimmune patients.

EFA's Essential Fatty Acids

Are essential because they occur outside the body and daily to stem the cravings of toxic fats you find in french fries, and potato chips. EFA's also help reduce obesity by reducing inflammation by balancing Omega 6 and Omega 3. The healthy ratio is 3:1, but with food preservatives using unhealthy Omega 6 as an ingredient in just about everything, the average North American has unhealthy ratios as high as 30:1 (see weight loss). Healthy EFA's changes the ratio of LDL's and HDL cholesterol significantly lowering risk of heart disease.

DHA - Docosahexaenoic acid found in supplements and is an omega-3 fatty acid.

EPA - Eicosapentaenoic acid found in supplements and is an omega-3 fatty acid.

ALA - Alpha Linolenic acid found in flaxseed oil and is an omega-3.

GLA - Gamma Linolenic acid is found in borage oil or primrose oil.

Oleic acid is an omega 9 found in olive oil and coconut oil.

Essential fatty acids are essential and without them you will die.

Ego

Ego blocks the truth and lives in belief. Belief closes your mind to see the truth, because if what you believe doesn't match what you hear, the information is blocked without consideration. Ego only cares about self, possessions and beliefs. Low vibration frequencies are that of ego, judgment, fear, resentment, jealousy, anger, rage, selfishness, possessions, hatred, war, and fear of the past, present, and future which serves to lower pH, overall health and potential.

Exercise

Has several benefits. It is a method of excreting toxins through sweat and movement and jarring of cells and lymph nodes. It feeds your cells with disease fighting oxygen, by increasing your lungs efficiency to exchange oxygen at the capillary level. Exercise also speeds up metabolism. It is also a mood elevator by releasing endorphins into the blood stream. Exercise for weight loss is best done in the morning which increase metabolism throughout the day. Advanced training is done using wind sprints off and on to maximize benefits. Patients with autoimmune shouldn't be doing vigorous exercise because it drains the adrenals and furthermore, muscles that are exercised creates permanent damage. Long distance running is not considered healthy because of stress on joints and critical nutrient levels that are not replaced with normal diets. People overweight, considered obese shouldn't be exercising at a high heart rate because it stresses the heart. They should wait until their weight is reduced to a safe level before they engage in jogging. Carbohydrate loading, like eating spaghetti, can be done just prior to a marathon to feed your cells during your run. It is thought that cardio increases your IQ by about 10% through higher concentrations of oxygen in your blood from a developed efficiency of oxygen exchange in the capillaries that improves with regular exercise.

Feminization of the Male

The disappearing male is about one of the most important, and least publicized issues facing North Americans. The young men born since the mid 80's have low sperm counts, are suffering from genital deformities and abnormalities. A higher percentage of this age group of males are A-sexual (not interested in females) or gay, when compared to previous generations. Researchers can see why. Estrogen mimickers (which is essentially estrogen) is found in everything from shampoo, sunglasses, meat and dairy products, carpet, cosmetics and baby bottles, they are called "hormone mimicking" or "endocrine disrupting" chemicals and they are damaging the most basic building blocks of human development. It starts with the mothers passing down abnormally high levels of these estrogens to their fetuses. The results are the feminization of girls at a younger age, with breasts developing years younger than previous generations. As an observer, you can watch television shows that psychologically embrace this abnormal transformation with the evermore presence of gay celebrities on sitcoms, gay marriages, the News, and Jay Leno. The normalization is confirmation of an agenda for population control that is achieving success. Doctors will notice there is an increase of infertility concerns with patients disappointed. The primary corrective measures are iodine, trace minerals, meal replacement, removing yourself from electronic smog that kills testosterone, eliminating statin drugs in favor of Olestyr, and hormone analysis by a bioidentical hormone specialist. Men should focus on a DHEA supplement and women a progesterone cream to balance out the excess toxic estrogens in the blood. The best solution is stop putting xenoestrogens particularly, and 75,000 chemicals in our products we use and discover ethics.

Food labeling facts

Do all you can to grow your own food and buy from farmers and organic growers that don't put pesticides in the soil.

- Low Calorie means it is sweetened with a chemical sweetner, which means it is fattening.

- The FDA currently has no limit on the amount of heavy metals allowed in foods, which is another reason we need to pull the plug on their authority.
- The "use of some organics" means that some ingredients are "not" in consumer products.
- GMO are so widespread that they have now have contaminated virtually the entire food supply. The estimate of contamination in the US is 93%, which is going to take more than their entire market value to compensate farmers and consumer lawsuits on the horizon under "tort law". Tort Law, is a body of rights, obligations, and remedies that is applied by courts in civil proceedings to provide relief for persons who have suffered harm. I believe that there are 6 major companies involved in GMO.
- Beware of GMOs in gluten-free foods, because gluten-free foods are usually made with genetically modified corn containing BT toxin a deadly insecticide.
- Non GMO does not mean certified organic non-GMO.
- Trans Fat Free does not mean free from trans-fats.
- All Natural doesn't mean anything at all so check for ingredients you don't recognize. We need proper labeling for average shoppers who don't have chemistry degrees.
- Kosher does not mean non-GMO.

Fluoride, Chlorine, Bromine

See nutrition on how these substances in our water are killing humans. Rat poison is fluoride and is used as an injectable blood thinner. It is being injected randomly to just about every patient over 40 at your hospital and is called Heparin. Don't take it, because it will hurt you on several levels, when a little aspirin will do!

Flu Shots

Make you 2x more likely to get the flu and knocks out your immune system for 90 days after taking it. I met patients who took the flu shot that gave them permanent autoimmune disease from the squalene contained, which is a neurotoxin circulating in your blood unable, because of a chromosome 6 gene weakness, to eliminate neurotoxins (see chap 3). You are more likely to get the flu for 90 days following taking it.

Geoengineering/ Chemtrails

People need to get aware about this harmful genocide happening to our planet and all forms of life. The aluminum in the aerosol being sprayed across our skies is raising the pH of the soil, killing the organisms that are responsible for transferring the nutrients from the soil to the plants. Within 5 years it is expected that organic food grown outdoors will no longer be possible. You can watch an episode from JesseVentura.net filming the planes and airports from where this geoengineering is happening across North America. Measured nano-particulate of aluminum increase 50,000% in the air following chemtrailing across the skies. The smaller the particulate the more harm to the respiratory system. Artificially induced snow is happening at 44F from chemtrails. There is insect decline, bees and bird population decline, and the extinction rate of species that is 10,000x more than natural that is currently happening since spraying began. A significant problem is looming with the "Venus Syndrome". It is the feedback loops of methane gas being released from the floor of the oceans creating man made "climategate" that is a consequence of chemtrails. To add to the chemtrail cocktail of nuclear waste of barium, strontium radiation that is interfering with our DNA by getting into our crops and runoff into our drinking water.

http://www.geoengineeringwatch.org/coast-to-coast-am-daily-march-13th-2013-geoengineering-threats/ There are 3 parts to this episode of March 13/13 that exposes the science behind geoengineering that talks about how it is creating and intensifying health issues, contributes to global warming, droughts, floods, bark falling off trees, crop failures and extreme weather. (Www.carnicominstitute.org w/ Dane Wigington). Haarp is another weapons system that is being used in conjunction with geoengineering you might want to investigate. Our governments are out of control and too many people who know about this, are saying oh well.

Gestational Diabetes

Is principally caused by an inflamed pancreas from GMO's. Ketchup, mayonnaise and 1000's of products contain the non life-sustaining poison that inflames organs. Probiotics, glutathione, tumeric, vitamin C, D, E are good anti-oxidants to lower inflammation and free radicals. Meal replacements and juicing will help with the nutrients. Be sure to take iodine to boost the baby's IQ during pregnancy. Taking iodine post pregnancy will accelerate the fat removal around the tummy and make you fertile for the next one. Massage in organic oil on your tummy to stop stretch marks from day one of your pregnancy.

It is not a sign of good health to be well adjusted to a sick society.

GMO or GE (genetically modified or engineered)

The originators of GMO found bacteria surviving in a chemical waste dump and put it in the food supply. They took the gene that allowed bacteria to survive and put it into soy beans. Soy crops drinks up Round Up pesticide and stores it in the food we are eating. Round Up is an antibacterial, antibiotic, anti-life formula that is sprayed on crops and is killing the soil of organisms. It is in the blood of pregnant women and the blood of fetuses. BT Corn has a little gene sized spray bottle containing a toxin that breaks open the stomachs of insects and kills them, and now it is sold at your grocery and creates holes in cells of humans and causes intestinal pain. The usual pain point first felt is the lower right side of your stomach.

You will be hearing a lot about Genetically Modified Food Organisms until GMO's go away. 91-93% of people polled in the US, want GMO's labeled and the US is one of the only countries in the world where it is not mandatory. GMOs, or genetically modified organisms, are plants or animals that have been genetically engineered with undesirable DNA from bacteria, viruses, plants and animals. Virtually all commercial GMOs are engineered to withstand direct application of herbicide and/or to produce an insecticide. It is the insecticide that is causing problems with your internal organs and digestive tract and having people dropping like flies dead these days. Despite biotech industry promises, GMO traits currently on the market offer decreased yields, nor any consumer benefit and does destroy the soil in which it is grown and of those who eat it.

¾ of North Americans don't know they are eating GMO every meal. 60% say they have never eaten GMO and 75% eat it everyday. Infant formulas contain genetically engineered ingredients such as corn, soy, sugar without being labeled. A new petition urges infant formula makers to phase out all GMOs from their infant formulas. We have better things to do than protest and petition an obvious crime against humanity. Poison on the Platter and Genetic Roulette are good documentaries to watch on the subject. GMO is done with cross breeding the worst Dna of species of animals with plants. 27 countries have banned GMO's and 50 countries require labeling. The Swiss, Italy, Greece, French, Polish and Austrians have also banned it. They were introduced into supermarkets without FDA approval by Monsanto "as safe", and independent lab tests are revealing shocking results. Lab rats have tumors all over their bodies and farm animals are falling over dying within 6 months of eating it. Humans are having their organs go into inflammation that are beginning to shut down after about 11 years of eating it. Tests have found that the protein from BT corn continues to reproduce poison toxins in your gut for days after you eat it. Insects that eat the corn have their stomachs explode and bees that come in contact with the pesticides this company makes are dying with their stomachs exploding as well. When the food is grown with pesticides applied to the soil, up to 90% of the cross section of nutrients doesn't make it out of that soil to the produce. The cycle of life is destroyed because the organisms that facilitate the transfer of life to your dinner table are dead and GMO only ramps up this horrifying equation.

Hundreds of thousands of farmers are committing suicide drinking the Roundup pesticide after Monsanto tricked farmers to convert their fields over to growing with a pesticide/GMO combination, and with lower yields they failed to make break-even and were bankrupt. The corporate farming interests are buying up bankrupt farmers at pennies on the dollar and aggressively taking over and growing this toxic substance. But the worst thing is that they are not only destroying the soil of organisms but also the nutrients through unsustainable farming techniques. They are running the soil into a brick wall so no one can farm it for decades after. There are key ingredients that are being depleted in the soil like potassium. 80% of everything you eat contains GMO which is an irritant in the digestive tract, is reducing sperm counts and shutting down organ function in humans.

Hungary ordered the burning of their GMO crops and Japan refuses to import anything that might contain GMO for their people. Millions are marching and protesting GMOs, and the media is ignoring the parades, as more and more studies come out proving the toxicity of the food for consumption by man or animal. Gluten free seems to indicate GMO-free food but not always. Gluten is a protein that your body has a hard time digesting. Over 95% of Soy and corn is GMO and this is a crop you need a Hazmut suit to pick. I believe that it will take generations and trillions of dollars to clean up the mess to reconvert 420 million of acres of farmland back to a natural state and restore the health of the soil.

A proposed law in Chile that would have allowed Monsanto to patent genetically modified seeds has resulted in a massive, spontaneous protest against GMOs and seed patents. Market analysts can't deny the fact that millions of awakening people are causing Monsanto share prices to go down and stay down. Natural Food Certifiers (NFC) recently announced it will no longer certify as kosher any foods or food brands that contain or use GMOs. Canola oil is GMO made with rape seed. Science research is rigged to avoid finding problems, but when they found serious problems they then dismissed them. Scientists refuse to research GMO because of threats to them and their families. What ethical science has found, is that in the 1st 90 days of rat lab tests found, organ damage, premature deaths and genetic mutations and tumors that deformed the tested animals that were grotesque to look at.

Below is the hierarchy of what appears to be a pathway of corruption. Checks and balances are ignored in the passage of GMO food from a lab of a chemical company to your dinner plate. The political system favors the company and not what is in the best interests of the people it serves. In waiting are the same people who own the pharmaceuticals and run your patient health. Vertical integration is making people sick and bankrupting families on a massive level. Look at this corrupted system of conflict of interest. Families cannot live in a system that runs like this:

Monsanto employee	Monsanto position	US Government position
Toby Moffett	Monsanto consultant	US Congressman (D)
Dennis DeConcini	Monsanto legal council	US Senator (D)
Margaret Miller	Chemical lab supervisor	Deputy Director of the FDA
Marcia Hale	Director Int'l Govt. Affairs	White House Senior Staff
Mikey Kantor	Member of Board	US Secretary of Commerce
Virginia Weldon	Vice Pres. Public Policy	White House CSA
Josh King	Director Int'l Govt. Affairs	White House Communications
David Beler	V.P. Govt. and Public Affairs	Al Gore Chief Policy Advisor
Carol Tucker-Foreman	Lobbyist for Monsanto	White House appointed Consumer Advocate
Linda Fisher	V.P. Govt. and Public Affairs	Deputy Admin of the EPA
Lidia Watrud	Manager, New Technologies	USDA, EPA
Michael Taylor	V.P. Public Policy	Deputy Commissioner, FDA
Hillary Clinton	Monsanto Council	First Lady, US Senator (D), Sec State
Roger Bleachy	Director, Monsanto	Director USDA NIFA
Islam Siddiqui	Monsanto Lobbyist	Agriculture Negotiator Trade Rep.
Clarence Thomas	Monsanto Council	US Supreme Court Judge
Donald Rumsfeld	Board of Directors	US Secretary of Defense
Anne Veneman	Board of Directors	US Secretary of Agriculture

Senators who voted against GMO labeling while not protecting the Bill of Rights, will be publicly shamed for selling out. Here's the list of the 71 senators that sided with Monsanto and not the will of the people. Make sure they don't get back in!! How about a recall to clean up this list. The only seats they deserve is in a cell.

Alexander (R-TN)	Ayotte (R-NH)	Baldwin (D-WI)	Barrasso (R-WY)
Baucus (D-MT)	Blunt (R-MO)	Boozman (R-AR)	Brown (D-OH)
Burr (R-NC)	Carper (D-DE)	Casey (D-PA)	Chambliss (R-GA)
Coats (R-IN)	Coburn (R-OK)	Cochran (R-MS)	Collins (R-ME)
Coons (D-DE)	Corker (R-TN)	Cornyn (R-TX)	Cowan (D-MA)
Crapo (R-ID)	Cruz (R-TX)	Donnelly (D-IN)	Durbin (D-IL)
Enzi (R-WY)	Fischer (R-NE)	Franken (D-MN)	Gillibrand (D-NY)
Graham (R-SC)	Grassley (R-IA)	Hagan (D-NC)	Harkin (D-IA)
Hatch (R-UT)	Heitkamp (D-ND)	Heller (R-NV)	Hoeven (R-ND)
Inhofe (R-OK)	Isakson (R-GA)	Johanns (R-NE)	Johnson (D-SD)
Johnson (R-WI)	Kaine (D-VA)	Kirk (R-IL)	Klobuchar (D-MN)
Landrieu (D-LA)	Lee (R-UT)	Levin (D-MI)	McCain (R-AZ)
McCaskill (D-MO)	McConnell (R-KY)	Menendez	(D-NJ) Moran (R-KS)

Nelson (D-FL)	Paul (R-KY)	Portman (R-OH)	Pryor (D-AR)
Risch (R-ID)	Roberts (R-KS)	Rubio (R-FL)	Scott (R-SC)
Sessions (R-AL)	Shaheen (D-NH)	Shelby (R-AL)	Stabenow (D-MI)
Thune (R-SD)	Toomey (R-PA)	Udall (D-CO)	Vitter (R-LA)
Warner (D-VA)	Warren (D-MA)	Wicker (R-MS)	

Ben & Jerry's will be non-GMO by the end of 2013, and while Chipotle's restaurants are working toward a non-GMO menu, they voluntarily started labeling in the meantime.

Gout

Is like diabetes but with a different organ. It is caused by an inflammation of the kidneys and or liver. Excess uric acid is the symptom of gout and leads to the formation of Kidney stones. I believe that uric acid is a symptom of poor diet like soft drinks and GMO. Eating food your body recognizes and cleansing and flushing stones from your kidneys and liver will get rid of gout. You can reduce the symptom of inflammation with glutathione and by drinking organic parsley tea. Chanca Piedra is called a stone crusher and you take 6 capsules a day for 2-4 weeks to dissolve 80% of kidney stones and 20% of stones in your liver. 3$ worth of parsley in a pot on boil for 20 minutes, later throw away the parsley, and drink a mug of the watery broth each day for 7 days. You should be on this water broth regularly for maintenance for the nutrients to rebuild your kidney's integrity. Expect to do Isacleanse and perhaps 6 of them, one every weekend for deep cellular cleansing until there are no further benefits, and perhaps glutathione and or oxygen for symptoms and meal replacement am and pm for cause. When you correct gout, you end up correcting a dozen other problems like weight loss due to inflamed kidneys and liver.

Source of inflammation can be either from exposure to toxic mold or malnutrition or toxins in your food or all 3, and it makes for a body that is out of balance. Fish oil contributes to gout, so you could try primrose oil instead. A sick liver's inability doesn't break down uric acid into separate carbon units is part of the reason for gout. Good to add selenium to your diet with iodine. Cherries prevent gout naturally.

Hepatitis

ALA or alpha lipoic acid intravenous (IV) to help with symptoms, is used for the acceleration in rebuilding of damaged livers. Because oxygen can kill viruses and bacteria, oxygen therapy should be considered to get rid of the virus that causes hepatitis. Vaccinations I don't think are necessary because of oxygen (see oxygen). The risks of hepatitis vaccinations are not worth it in my opinion from the horror stories I am reading about and talking to victims who take vaccinations.

Herpes and Genital Warts

Cold sores and genital sores come out when you are stressed, dehydrated, malnourished, and tired for those that have been exposed to the virus that is in your body. Because both are viruses they can be killed with oxygen therapy, but because they hide in healthy cells, it can take a long maintenance dose to achieve, if at all. Flare ups caught early can be eliminated quickly in a day with h2o2 hydrogen peroxide food grade, if your gut is healthy enough to tolerate 15 drops 3x/day, an hour before food or 2 hours after food. Drink a lot of water when you start to feel symptoms coming on. Be careful taking this product because it reacts to food and drink other than water. When h2o2 takes out candida, it can create a toxic overload in your gut. Flushing with water is necessary and more of it if you feel a headache coming on. Absorption of toxins occur in your gut so flushing is necessary following oxygen use. More testing needs to be done to confirm conclusively for permanent success using oxygen treatment on both viruses. The same type of stabilized oxygen with 11% ozone daily might be enough to hold off outbreaks. The lysine amino acid sold in 1000mg 1x/day, from a health food store, helps stem the frequency and severity of outbreaks of herpes and genital warts.

Hypertension

Hypertension is a symptom of inflammation. The primary cause of hypertension is a mal-functioning sick liver that is plugged with gallstones, with fatty deposits from a history of food and beverage choices that were toxic (chapter 4). The secondary cause is of broad spectrum mal-nourishment that leads to inflammation throughout your body from compromised cellular repair. Nitric oxide treats the symptom but not the cause of hypertension.

IBS

A healthy gut should be 85% good bacteria for digestion and 15% of the bad kind that make up gut flora. When the balance is out of ratio, you will begin to have a yeast infection in your gut. It is caused by poor diet as well as from taking antibiotics and GMO's.

A symptom of IBS is, carbon dioxide expanding and creating pain in your stomach and is perpetuated with foods like sweets, beer, bread, pastry, wheat and HFCS. Passing gas that doesn't smell and lower abdominal pain are your best tests to confirm the problem of IBS. The fastest way to take IBS out is with oxygen, using h2o2 food grade drops in a glass of water from a health food store. You start out with 3 drops 3x daily and you can quickly ramp it up day to day as you can tolerate the toxins from the die-off of anaerobic cells. The bad bacteria can make you feel sick. The symptom is called Herxheimer's effect, which is a form of toxic shock, so be careful when taking oxygen. The good bacteria will remain and you can accelerate the process with probiotic supplements to repopulate with good bacteria to correct IBS. Other ways of helping IBS or giving your gut a chance to heal is taking a pill called "digest IBS and there are Chinese herbs that break down the sugar of your food before it gets to the intestines where it becomes fuel for the yeast infection. With both methods, they are not so effective compared to using oxygen, and you want to take probiotics and digestive enzymes to speed up digestion and make it more efficient. Antibiotics, steroids, birth control pills, synthetic hormones, food toxins destroy good bacteria. These are just a sample of what can kill off the good bacteria, and inhibit your body's ability to fight off bad bacteria. A healthy gut is important. Half of your immune system, your central nervous system and your nutrient absorption exists there. Being disease and obese-free depends on a healthy gut. And I believe that a large part of mental illness and dementia originates from your gut. Taking oxygen by IV is expensive but gets concentration in your blood without feeling that sick taste. A new method that mixes aloe vera with h2o2 (food grade) helps your body tolerate a high dose and get fast conclusive results. The problem with candida is getting a high enough dose of oxygen and just about everything you eat antagonizes the condition with GMO's sugar and any alcohol. Specialists are dismissing patients who have severe cases of IBS, which is a misdiagnosis. Aloe vera gel in a glass of an ounce or two

3x/day is so helpful and immediate for symptoms of IBS from a health food store, for symptoms. The time is now to open up a health food store or organic restaurant, perhaps Italian?

Infertility

Some quick areas to focus on is low iodine in women. Iodine is the most important supplement in critical deficiency, along with trace vitamin deficiencies. Iodine should be taken double strength daily, if you drink municipal tap water and you are female. The secondary causes of infertility are low levels of 60 trace minerals found in the bottom of the seabed located in Utah and from low vitamin E. Hormone analysis can help too, to make sure progesterone levels are back up after following taking the pill that stops pregnancy. For men cortisol is the stress hormone that is the polar opposite to Testosterone. It blocks the Testosterone hormone. The estrogen mimickers from plastics raise obesity and lowers Testosterone levels. Wifi, smart meters in your home and electronics kill sperm counts and GMO's are said to cause infertility. Eugenics is now called "planned parenthood". Alcohol eats testosterone.

Law of attraction

The movie The Secret was misleading because of one important piece of information missing in their message is that, "what you manifest must be in alignment with your soul and your soul contract here on earth", otherwise you won't attract it. Law of attraction is best achieved when you are helping others and not yourself.

Leptin

Acts on receptors in the hypothalamus of the brain. Leptin is a hormone made by fat cells which helps to regulate the storage of fat. When leptin increases as the result of a mold exposure/autoimmune response, and MSH (alpha melanocyte stimulating hormone) decreases, people become overweight and weight loss is difficult even with diet and exercise. Lab mice treated, lost their excess fat and returned to normal body weights. Leptin itself was co-discovered in 1994.

Leukemia

The primary cause of leukemia is the low natural occurring element of arsenic in microscopic amounts of parts per billion in your blood.

Lyme Disease and Chronic Lyme

Both are curable but are nasty. Lyme disease is bacteria spread from the bite of a tic and is at epidemic proportions mostly across the northern US and across the southern part of Canada. The Western Blot test for Lyme is only done in the US, at a cost of about 300-400$ and is only about 50% accurate. The test for Lyme in Canada is only 5% accurate or 95% inaccurate. The test isn't really needed because of unreliability. If a week or 2 (about 25 cents) of h2o2 hydrogen peroxide doesn't work or improve symptoms or bring on a Herxheimer's reaction from spirochete die-off, then you probably haven't got Lyme disease. Pretreatment with 10 days of Actos Rx, a diabetic drug, and a non-amylose diet arrests the symptom of Herxheimer's. The after-bite is radial in nature and looks like a bulls-eye with red inflammation. If you catch it early in the first couple of weeks, antibiotics works effectively, but if you don't the spirochete burrows into your cells beyond the reach of antibiotics where treatment for a much longer time of perhaps 6-12 months might be necessary. Oxygen works better than antibiotics, but dose maximum might be only 24 drops a day for an extended period past 30 days.

The Chronic Lyme patients on the other hand will have devastating effects similar to autoimmune symptoms. Antibiotics or better, oxygen can take out the bacteria only to an extent where tolerance of Herxheimer's will warrant. That takes time and patience, but oxygen will be faster, more effective and done at a fraction of the cost than using antibiotics. Where bacteria has been removed and symptoms of illness persist or worsen, you no longer have Lyme disease, but chronic Lyme disease. Chronic Lyme is not Lyme disease but autoimmune disease or properly called, Biotoxin Illness. The DNA blood test on chromosome 6 subtype 52b and a few other subtypes can be confirmed with the HLA-dr test. The government has ignored Lyme disease and Chronic Lyme disease. It is believed to have originated from the biological warfare labs of Plum Island, off Lyme Connecticut. It is being moved to Manhattan Kansas.

Magnesium

Regulates 300 enzymes and reduces inflammation helping muscle and nerve function. Helps prevent artery hardening and with the elimination of gallstones by softening them.

Malaria

A cure for malaria was brought to Africa about 10 years ago and the product was primarily made of peptides from colostrum from cows and was curing villages of the disease within a day and the same product was working on AIDS patients within a week. The doctors were shot dead in the head and the rest left abruptly. This product is still available in the US. Because malaria is a parasitic organism, oxygen therapy will work as well.

Mammograms

Are ineffective and give you a 1000x more radiation than having a chest X-ray according to the chairman of the Cancer Prevention Coalition. There are too many false positives, about 40% of all that are done. It is thought that mammograms cause more breast cancer than they save. Cancer from radiation is hard to cure because it causes cellular mutation that is far worse than a case of cystic breast disease. Breast cancer and cystic breast disease are caused primarily by low iodine and to a lesser extent, estrogen mimickers. Progesterone prescribed by your doctor daily postmenopausal or on the last 15 days of your cycle should sop up the mess of estrogen mimickers and all should stop buying non-organic underarm deodorant, laundry detergent, and avoid plastics where you can.

Massage

Massage removes spasm from your body which allows for sleep debt to be released. When you store sleep your body is in spasm and that is unhealthy. Following a massage you need to sleep otherwise the spasm will stay in your body. Massage increases circulation and releases pockets of toxic stored energy, similar to yoga. It is best to have a drink of water following a treatment to eliminate toxins released by treatment from working the muscles.

Meat

Organic beef and chicken, two of the most popular meats consumed. Chickens are being grown in cages where they are not allowed to move and are being fed food that isn't part of their normal diet. That torture of the chicken is passed along as low Life Force energy into the meat and eggs to consumers.

One of the ingredients being fed chickens is Asarone. In the dictionary arsenic is poison, one of the main ingredients of Asarone. It is the king of poisons because it is tasteless and odorless. It is used in rat poison, weed killer and in glass manufacturing. Each time you eat chicken, you eat arsenic. That's right, arsenic is used as feed to increase weight and improve the color of the chicken meat. No studies were done to see the effects for safety but it doesn't take a 10 year old to figure out the effects. When the European Union did the first tests, they banned arsenic in chicken feed immediately, but it is still being fed to chickens in the rest of the world. Small amounts of arsenic consumed cause bladder, lung, kidney, and colon cancer. It hurts the immune, neurological and endocrine systems, can lead to partial paralysis and diabetes and a decline in brain functions. Chicken that is non-organic are dropped into vats of industrial strength chlorine and then moved into a vat of salt to disguise the taste of the toxic chlorine. The chlorine is almost as toxic as the arsenic.

Chicken excrement is then made into pellets containing this arsenic and along with GMO corn and alfalfa and is fed to cattle to fatten them up in the last 60 days of a cow's life before slaughter. By toxifying the cow's liver with arsenic and this unnatural diet, the cattle balloon up on average of 400 lbs. They have trouble standing up and start frothing at the mouth and their eyes have trouble focusing, before they are killed or are brought in dead with a front end loader for butchering. Watch Food Inc on Youtube.com for some graphic images. Needless to say, the Life Force energy of the meat is poor at best and the toxic meat is passed on to humans. The livers can't be salvaged, because the organ is loaded with puss. These chemicals in chicken and beef are pervasive, and are known to cause cancer, cardiovascular disease, type 2 diabetes, mental impairment, miscarriage, and other serious human health issues. 80% of all antibiotics are used on factory farms to keep unnatural diets and lifestyle of herds alive long enough for slaughter.

Menstrual Cramps

Go away with 5-10,000 iu of vitamin D within 30 minutes, and taking EFA's for a couple of months also seems to help with cramps.

Mental Illness/ Dementia

Can be the hardest illness to overcome. The human mind is like a black box and people react differently to signals and stimulation. Shutting down the mind with drugs desensitizes your mind to stimulation and life's signals. The more powerful the drug the more desensitized you become. This might be helpful temporarily but for the long term there are many sources or layers possible that can be out of balance that can be corrected to eliminate mental illness. Getting rid of all inflammation, disease and obesity is of primary importance. I believe that you should first reduce inflammation in the gut with the IBS protocol, increase hormones to a level of a 30 year old, and detoxing the liver are the main elements to focus on. Your nutrient density and bioavailability is important so follow the "Do's and Don'ts" of chapter 2. Taking niacin for schizophrenia seems to help. Reiki or crystal healing to align chakras and to eliminate negative energies worked profoundly on 19 out of 20 people with one session of an hour.

The main cause of mental illness is caused by exposure to the presence of neurotoxins from exposure to toxic environmental mold in your home and at work, so focus on detoxing and chelation. I hear of great success stories using this strategy.

Euphoria comes from a healthy body. Mental illness comes from a sick body that is inflamed and out of balance over a long period of time at the cellular level. Mental illness is acquired through insidious cellular degeneration malnourishment and from toxins in what you eat, drink and the environment you live and how you deal with those toxins over years. Luck comes from hard work delivered by means of a healthy body. The body is an instrument that when it is not operating properly will let you down emotionally. It is not hard to comprehend how devastating our food and water and consumer products have become. The normal was of 100 years ago when 1 in 100,000 kids had autism and now 1 in 50 do, and to some extent, for everyone who take a vaccination today. Going back to normal requires the elimination of the 75,000 chemicals that have been added to the food chain. You do need to surround yourself and fill your days with things, ideas, people, employment, that stimulate and arouse passion. Better to have a short life doing what you enjoy. Follow your bliss like a child would. It is the children that should be teaching the parents to follow their bliss and the parents should be there to teach survival.

Mercury Silver Teeth Fillings

One drop of mercury in a large pond would consider it contaminated, yet a lot of North Americans have that much mercury as fillings in their mouths. Every time you chew your food a small quantity gets released into your digestion. It is cumulative and one of the most toxic substances on earth. I have read that the electronic smog from frequencies being circulated in our homes is also responsible for releasing trace amounts of mercury from dental fillings.

Microwave Danger!

The science project that circulated around the internet involved boiling a cup of water in a microwave and on a stove. After cooling, the water is added to 2 identical plants. One plant fed by water from the microwave and the other plant from the stove. The plant watered from the microwave, shriveled up within a 9 days and the plant watered from the stove thrived.

Microwaves corrupts the DNA in the food so the body can't recognize it. The body wraps the microwaved food in fat cells or tries to eliminate it. Think of all the mothers heating up baby formula. The microwave destroys the nutrients in the oven and rearranges the DNA so that the body doesn't recognize the formula. There is the story of the nurse in Canada that warmed up blood to body temperature for a blood transfusion in a microwave and it killed the patient dead. But Authority says that microwaves are safe? Another story that didn't make it to the News.

10 REASONS TO THROW OUT YOUR MICROWAVE OVEN

1 - Continually eating food cooked in a microwave oven causes long term permanent brain damage by shorting out electrical impulses in the brain by depolarizing or demagnetizing the brain tissue.
2 - The human body can't metabolize or break down the unknown byproducts created in microwaved food.

3 - Male and female hormone production is shut down and or altered by continuous eating of microwaved foods.

4 - The effects of microwaved food byproducts are residual long term, and permanent within the body.

5 - Minerals, vitamins, and nutrients of all microwaved food is reduced or destroyed so that the body gets little benefit. The body can't absorb the cooked food that can't be broken down for digestion.

6 - The minerals in vegetables are turned into cancer causing free radicals

7 - Microwaved foods cause stomach and intestinal cancer growths.

8 - Eating microwaved food causes cancer cells to increase in your blood.

9 - Food from it, causes loss of memory, concentration emotional stability and intelligence from depolarization.

10-Causes immune system deficiencies by lymph gland and blood serum changes.

Youtube.com "effects of microwave"

Throw out your microwave, and use a toaster oven. The use of microwave ovens subliminally controls your mind and it has been proven.

Misinformation

The problem we face of getting useful information to people, is that the "reliable" sources of information are really sources of "misinformation". Just about everything that is being introduced as "official" policy on getting healthy, is in contradiction of what you should do to get and stay healthy. Every idea or advancement in health today reported in the media and on government websites are introducing and intensifying causes of inflammation. At the same time, there are more and more restrictions to access to the products that reduce inflammation. For example, supplements, super foods, cleanses for the liver, oxygen (h2o2), and personal freedoms are being removed aggressively by our governments (the G20 in Toronto was a perfect example). The restrictions to access are the essentials that cure the imbalances that lead to inflammation, and disease. Many of us are finding this disturbing and it is going largely unnoticed by too many. Remedies are being removed by stealth like a python squeezing the life out of a rabbit. Most don't know it, because decline in health and strategy is implemented gradually and it's imperceptible. Agenda 21 involves injection of more and more sophisticated poison into food and water, and the extraction of nutrients out of food, using pasteurization, radiation, pesticides, and processing. When you raise inflammation in the body, it creates a malaise, apathy and a dumbing down across the board of the participants, and is done especially with toxins in our drinking water which has a disturbing toxic effect that makes the brain go numb.

The NEWS MEDIA are just parrots that support the parade of misinformation with reports that there is no difference between organic and non-organic. Organic is regular normal food where the nutrients are present typical of spinach 60 years ago before pesticides. The science behind pesticides is that it is used to kill the organisms in the ground that cut off the transfer of nutrients from the soil to the plant. The live organisms in the soil make the nutrients bioavailable to the plants, and without live organisms in the ground, the cycle of life starves the plant up to 90% of every nutrient that makes up the profile of our produce. This is a major cause of obesity and inflammation, because you have to eat 8 salads of spinach to match 1 ordinary salad from your backyard. The science doesn't lie and the truth can only prevail only with a media. Who owns the media and who benefits. Follow the money.

News by the way, stands for information from the north, east, west and south and the News today is just propaganda absent of fact. It has been proven that if an audience hears something 3x, they will just about believe anything, without necessarily understanding. This is the 100 monkey theory, or some call it the "sheeple effect".

The GOVERNMENT is advising you to stay out of the midday sun, wear a shirt, slap on suntan lotion regularly, take vaccinations, take only 400 ui of vitamin D and now 2000 ui of vitamin D, drink 8 glasses of municipal water, wash your hands with anti bacterial soap and wear sunglasses. All this advice hurts people and leads to inflammation, disease, depression and obesity. The government approved aspartame which is a cytoxin poison and its origin is from the feces of ecoli, a very dangerous bacteria for human life approved by our government and aspartame and the artificial sweetner under different names is in 6000 products.

MMS - MiracleMineral.org

Jim Humble, a brilliant scientist founded the miracle mineral supplement called MMS. Chlorine Dioxide is the mineral supplement that is a powerful antioxidant that fights disease by targeting anaerobic cells. It is more selective at removing anaerobic cells than, h_2o_2 hydrogen peroxide (food grade). All oxygen are effective at taking disease and cancer out of your body, and by reducing symptoms of inflammation, autism, MS, and autoimmune as well. Buy Jim's book, the FDA is currently after him and other cures, like hydrogen peroxide. You can support Jim and his fight against tyranny.

Monsanto

Now affectionately referred to as Mon-satan, seems to be in the business of evil from what I read from every source I've come across. They are the company that came out with Agent Orange, and this is the company that said DDT and PCB's were safe. Now they are in the business of bringing death to your dinner plate on a scale of destruction to the planet that will take trillions of dollars to rectify and a generation or two to restore the earth where it is grown on, back to normal.

Morgellons

Morgellons starts with relentless itching, stinging or biting sensations from organic "bugs" for lack of a better name. It is now being referred to as the "GMO/chemtrail disease", because evidence from lab tests have confirmed the source of this disease in North America. Cotton-like inorganic fibers appear on the body with no reasonable explanation. Skin rash develops along with lesions that will not heal. Many sufferers report string-like fibers of varying color popping out through the skin lesions. These fibers can be black, white, red or blue. Others report organic black specks falling from their bodies that litter their sheets and bathrooms. A variety of bugs and worms begin to find their way out of the body through the lesions. Other symptoms include hair loss, debilitating chronic fatigue, hard nodules beneath the skin, and joint pain. Morgellons is a manmade disease that is at pandemic levels in Canada and the US and there are more reports in California than anywhere else.

It is being spread by chemtrails, GMO's and processed food, and by vaccinations. Morgellons is made up of complex pathogens or organic and inorganic configuration of fibers, fungus, viruses, heavy metals and bacteria. Morgellons whatever it is…is cloaked from the immune system. It's different and it's dangerous. Patients who are going to their doctors are being referred to psychiatric institutions, some without option! The doctors are ignoring symptoms and the ones who take symptoms seriously are being threatened with medical license removal, so be warned.

One remedy: We have been able to get it under control fast by sipping an 1/8th of a teaspoon of Borax (laundry detergent) dissolved in a half to a full liter/quart of water and sipped throughout the day. Caution: Borax is somewhat toxic and deposits in your liver over time, but for those who take it, the benefits outweigh the health concerns. You should wash your clothes with Borax "mule". It comes in a green cardboard box. I hope the government doesn't take that off the shelf too. Externally rubbing bentonite clay on your body, allows the skin to open up and fibers spill out "in droves", and taking 15 drops/day of h2o2 food grade from a health food store in a glass of water, 1 hour before food or 2 hours after eating. Nothing but water can be consumed during this time.

You can spray your house by a hand spray with a mixture of 3 tbsp. of tetra sodium EDTA (ethylenediaminetetraacetic acid) as a chelating agent, used to decrease the reactivity of metal ions that may be present, and 4-5 tbsp. of ammonia with water (500ml/1/2qt). The mites or whatever they are, die and appear as black spots on your skin. They are alive and like your bathroom ceiling and move throughout your house. You can spray it in your bed and watch the organic black spots of dead organisms appear within minutes, where ever you feel them itch. You should wash the solution through your hair and doing that stops your hair from falling out in 5-7 days. For cats and dogs, they need to drink the Borax solution and wash their fir with the tetra sodium sodium/water solution. A scientist has come forward and disclosed that he worked on the development of Morgellons and "the intention was of spraying it on humans - the enemy". He later regretted helping with the development when he later found out that it is being sprayed on US citizens under the geoengineering program. Some research can be found at: Carnicom.com. These people's lives are in danger for coming forward by the US government, and CIA.

Motivation

Comes from energy, energy is real, it can be seen, it can be felt and it can be measured. Sex is the most healing means there is to man with self-love from the heart. Orgasm from the heart, along with self-love and self-respect is most powerful means to expand the soul, your aura, and to your experience bliss. Bliss is achieved with intimate feelings + orgasm and honesty, but you are left with emptiness with the absence of feelings.

MRSA
(Methicillin-Resistant Staphylococcus Aureus)

Is mainly caused by low iodine. Liver cleanses and high density meal replacements help. Iodine in the thyroid works like ultra violet light killing bacteria as blood passes through. The best iodine is matched with iodide, with selenium, B2 added for activation. www.staph-infection-resources. com where you can find a book that tells you how to rid yourself of MRSA step by step in detail. While you are waiting for the book, start taking iodine from your health food store and stay on it for life. The FDA might burn this book too?

MS

There are 2 types of MS both caused by neurotoxins in the blood from mold. One is the vascular type, which is starving veins of vital blood flow to muscles of oxygen and nutrients. The most common vein is the juggler that gets choked off confirmed by ultrasound. The procedure to correct, is a stint or a series of stints to open up blood restriction and it isn't always limited to the juggler vein. People who want the "stint" operation to open up collapsed veins are going to Mexico, Poland and India. I believe that the veins are collapsing due to an innate immune system response to due to autoimmune exposure to mold. It is the only element of health that deforms the body on a physical level. Our government is determined to withhold this successful MS solution by whatever excuse they can muster, with the aid of the media propaganda machine.

The other type of MS is Biotoxin related. This less common type of MS is the science behind autoimmune. It happens by means of an innate immune system response to neurotoxins in the blood, resulting in damage to the body that takes out layers of the myelin sheath that then shorts out electrical signals to the muscles from the brain. The solution for MS has been found and no further research is necessary for widespread implementation.

The one solution for vascular MS using a stint was found in the 1930's and the doctor was laughed off the public stage by the Medical Association and the media. The doctor subsequently dropped his work to live out a normal life. Those notes were found in a library during the 1960's by a doctor and were reopened for further investigation. What he found, filled in a few holes when he presented his findings, and the doctor had the same reaction as the previous doctor, but ridicule by a more polished organization. It was either promote his findings and risk his career or put it back on the shelf.

Dr Zamboni enters the stage from Italy, in 2007 with his wife ill with MS, desperate to find a solution for her, he stumbles across the research from the doctors of the 1930's and 1960's and he applies the modern equipment of ultrasound to confirm what he finds in the libraries. He confirms a lack of blood flow in his wife's juggler vein and sees only benefit to open up a vein that should be allowing the flow of blood and proves the hypothesis with a successful implant of a stint on his wife. The stint implant, is a day surgery procedure while the patient is awake and low and behold, symptoms of MS are virtually gone the same day. Light physio following to stimulate deteriorated muscles from lack of blood flow is a minor issue. He wants to tell the world and why not? News gets around the world and I am wondering how they are going to not offer this treatment to everyone? How? They stage an event in Mexico of someone dying, the media kicks in and the whole method for cure collapses and it is soon swept under the carpet by the medical association and the media. Poof! What happened?

Note: Statin drugs lead to symptoms of MS because it dissolves the myelin sheath that protects the nerves from shorting out to the muscles. Statin drugs reduce cholesterol and are dangerous, because cholesterol is the essential building block of cellular life.

Muscular Dystrophy

It is caused by a selenium deficiency. A few other lesser important supplements should be taken as well, iodine and meal replacement and trace minerals for cellular repair from your health food store. Your body operates like a symphony. You must avoid GMO and avoid gluten. Dystrophy means faulty nutrition. I heard that Jerry Lewis who used to run the telethon was relieved of his duties under a gag order when he discovered this way to beat MD. Millions of $$ are being wasted fund raising for a cause that has already been found instead of getting this nutrient to the people that need it. Perhaps that is why over 90% of monies collected don't make it to where the solution might be discovered. (Solution means Cure in laymen's terms)

Nitric Oxide (NO)

Works well at reducing high blood pressure symptoms but not the cause. From diabetes to hypertension, cancer to drug addiction, stroke to intestinal motility, memory and learning disorders to septic shock, sunburn to anorexia, male impotence to tuberculosis, there is probably no pathological condition where nitric oxide does not play an important role. Sun tanning helps with nitric oxide production naturally.

Nuclear

I read an article that stated whatever happens in the animal population happens to humans. Alligators in swamps downwind from nuclear plants are forgetting how to reproduce in Florida. Radiation confuses DNA in another report. Dairy farms around reactors have the highest rate of diabetes.

ORMEs Orbitally Rearranged Monatomic Elements,

Don't heal you but it cleans up the oxidation on the end caps of your DNA. Every cell then is rejuvenated. I tried various types and didn't sense any improvement personally, but for some they see improvements in cognitive function. There are different types that focus on the body, the heart and one for the mind. Isagenix has a "product B" supplement that helps to preserve the ends of your chromosomes from deteriorating associated with aging.

Osteoarthritis

Is an autoimmune disease caused by environmental toxic mold from where you live or work (see chapter 3). Inflammation is a result of firing a muscle to work. When a muscle is used there is a small amount of muscle repair following that use similar to a weight lifter following a workout. Where there is increased blood flow there are increased neurotoxins which are then tagged by the innate immune system that takes out the neurotoxin as it should, but along with it a small sample of tissue, bone, cartilage goes with it from the inflamed area. People with autoimmune shouldn't be exercising because you are actually destroying the muscles most used over time. That is why knee and hip replacement along with arthritis in the hands is prevalent. 24% of the population have the gene for autoimmune on chromosome 6 of the innate immune system, that reabsorb the neurotoxin over and over as chronic fatigue. To compound the problem of autoimmune, 35% of homes in North America cause symptoms of autoimmune/biotoxin illness due to mold present from flawed building codes that put residents in homes living in plastic bags with steep temperature gradients to the temperatures outside of their homes.

Osteoporosis

Occurs in a malnourished, toxic, hormone deficient, inflamed acidic body over time. It is the acidic blood trying to preserve its pH 7.0, leaching minerals out of your bones as a consequence. I cured Osteoporosis by rebalancing the 5 elements of health with high density nutrient meal replacements and organic fruits, vegetables and juicing along with supplements, like chlorella, spirulina, alfalfa, EFA's essential fatty acids, a triple dose of iodine from a health food store and I stopped drinking and bathing in tap water with fluoride and chlorine. Bio identical hormones seemed to have the biggest impact, next to avoiding living and working in a toxic mold free environment. I also flushed my liver of gallstones and parasites and it helps for anyone who wants to get rid of Osteo. I took 10,000 iu of vitamin D and added a tablet of high quality tumeric daily. You should be able to see improvement in 30 days and be free of Osteoporosis in 120 days. Replacing minerals with calcium is not a solution to Osteoporosis. It has a bio availability rate of close to 1% and the other 99% is unhealthy and deposits in your body where it is not needed.

Coral calcium has a much higher bioavailability but taking calcium treats the symptom and not the cause, about is as effective as pushing rope.

Osteoporosis is a common problem among the +50 crowd and especially in women. I had osteoporosis so bad that I broke my femur twice while I was walking and I didn't know how I did it. The major cause was autoimmune. The doctors were shocked months later looking at my x-rays. I cured myself of Osteoporosis using the 5 elements of the Matrix and today I have bone mass of someone 20 years younger than my peers. (more info in chapter 1)

Ovarian Cancer

Like prostate cancer, I believe the primary cause is unopposed estrogen sourced from BPA and BPS found in plastics non-organic underarm deodorant, laundry detergent, and eating meat injected with Bovine growth hormone. These all contain estrogen mimickers that are powerful toxic substances to the human body even found in trace amounts. Mothers are passing down these dangerous xenoestrogens down to their babies. I would suggest going to a bioidentical hormone specialist for an evaluation of overall hormone levels to supplement and monitor. For the financially desperate I would order Progest 50, off the internet to counteract the excess unopposed estrogen. For those cycling you apply the formula on the last 15 days of your cycle and for those who are post cycle you take progesterone daily.

Oxygen

There are 2 types of oxygen, one is therapeutic and reactive to take out disease, and the other type is stabilized oxygen to enhance health you can take with food with 11% ozone O3. It is a natural and non toxic bacteriocide, virucide and fungicide you can take everyday. Another awesome method of getting oxygen into the body to kill diseased cells is h2o2, by intravenous. Hydrogen Peroxide (must be food grade from a health food store). Look for 29% or 35% concentration and the drops are added to a glass of inert distilled water or regular water mixed with the drops sitting over night (read One Minute Cure). Oxygen helps the body metabolize nutrients, lowers inflammation, increases energy, pH and subsequently IQ. Almost all disease is anaerobic. Disease cannot thrive in an oxygen rich body. Oxygen can annihilate super bugs and the inflammation that cause cancer. Antibiotics are virtually redundant today.

Hyperbaric chambers are great for getting oxygen into the cells using a capsule of high pressure atmosphere you sit in administered by a skilled trained operator for an hour of breathing oxygen from a tank. The oxygen gets into the cells under pressure and relieves inflammation. Cardio exercise is a method of getting oxygen into the cells to prevent disease.

OZONE O3 is another source of powerful therapeutic oxygen done intravenously. Aother type of oxygen is using MMS. All methods takes out the anaerobic cells (disease and cancer) but the MMS method targets the cells more specifically and is able to leave good aerobic cells in tact. It is a 2 part system of drops mixed before water is added to your glass. The FDA and North American governments are trying to bust distributors and they have the originator Jim Humble in court today to financially ruin him. Please help him. The public that are aware of his successful product are waging a campaign to support his science. Hydrogen Peroxide Food Grade 29% is also under attack today by the Canadian Government trying to get it off the shelves sold at health food stores. The Canadian government already reduced the concentration down from 35% to 29%, and is asking health food stores to take it off the shelves and hide in cupboards. 1$ of h2o2 typically removes cancer for anyone. Oxygen is close to having a 100% success rate at curing cancer. I used it to help me cure my cancer. Stabilized oxygen is just for maintenance and doesn't have the concentration to work as effectively as the other 3.

Long term use of therapeutic oxygen should be limited to small doses because oxygen is caustic.

Most disease isn't really a disease but merely a symptom of an imbalance and can't be corrected with oxygen. Oxygen is really a quick fix to buy time until you get imbalances corrected. The oxygen treatment doesn't really help autoimmune, osteoporosis, or MS patients to cure the cause of disease but helps with symptoms of inflammation. A maintenance dose of oxygen can be used as a preventative method for disease, taken 8-10 drops in the morning, by killing virus, bacteria, candida, and chasing the herpes virus and genital warts viruses when they poke their head out. This is a simple, inexpensive and very broad spectrum healing process that many feel could force a complete overhaul of the medical industry. AIDS, herpes, hepatitis, Epstein Barr, cytomeglaovirus and other lipid envelope virus are readily destroyed by aggressive "hyper-oxygenating" the patient's blood with ozone. The problem with taking oxygen is getting up to concentration for effectiveness without feeling sick. It is awful to ingest, but there is a proprietary mixture available of aloe vera and h2o2 food grade which allows for higher concentrations. Oxygen is toxic when concentrated, but when diluted to therapeutic levels for h2o2 of 0.5% or less, it is not only non-toxic but extremely beneficial.

DOSAGE:

Use the dosages listed in the chart with 6 ounces of distilled or purified water. When reaching higher dosages 8-10oz. water should be used.

Take on an empty stomach, 1 hour before a meal and at least 2 hours after a meal. If your stomach gets upset at any level, stay at that level of dosage, or go back one level.

NOTE: Candida victims may need to start at 1 drop 3 times per day because of potential sensitivity.

DOSAGE SCHEDULE for undiluted 29% Canada /35% USA for h2o2
1st day, use 9 drops (3 drops, 3 times/day)
2nd day, use 12 drops (4 drops, 3 times/day)
3rd day, use 15 drops (5 drops, 3 times/day)
4th day, use 18 drops (6 drops, 3 times/day)
5th day, use 21 drops (7 drops, 3 times/day)
6th day, use 24 drops (8 drops, 3 times/day)
7th day, use 27 drops (9 drops, 3 times/day)
8th day, use 30 drops (10 drops, 3 times/day)
9th day, use 36 drops (12 drops, 3 times/day
10th day, use 42 drops (14 drops, 3 times/day)
11th day, use 48 drops (16 drops, 3 times/day)
12th day, use 54 drops (18 drops, 3 times/day
13th day, use 60 drops (20 drops, 3 times/day)
14th day, use 66 drops (22 drops, 3 times/day)
15th day, use 72 drops (24 drops, 3 times/day
16th day, use 75 drops (25 drops, 3 times/day)

For more serious illness try to stay at 20-25 drops, 3 times per day for 3 weeks. Next graduate down to 20-25 drops, 2 times per day until the problem is taken care of. 20 drops or more is suggested to have real impact. When free of illness, you may taper off by taking:

25 drops once every other day, 4 times
25 drops once every third day for 2 weeks
25 drops once every fourth day for 3 weeks
A good maintenance would be 10 - 15 drops per week

Oxygen buffered in aloe vera is a potent delivery of the molecule into your body to fight disease.

Oxidative Medicine Foundation is supporting clinical hydrogen peroxide food grade IV (intravenous injections). For doctor referrals write or call: P.O. Box 13205, Oklahoma City, OK 73113, 1-(405) 478-4266. No doctors are allowed to admit they can cure anything, but it is my opinion that this will for disease where virus, bacteria is the cause and will help with inflammation and actually take out cancer which is a symptom of excessive inflammation. Ozone and h2o2 therapies are considered cutting edge alternative health care protocols for treating a wide range of chronic illnesses including, cancer, AID's, hepatitis and tumors. This is information that the FDA would prefer you didn't read.

Ozone blood treatment

Ozone overcomes the AIDS virus by a different process than usually attempted with drugs. Instead of burdening the liver and immune system with toxic substances, ozone simply oxidizes the molecules in the shell of the AIDS virus and also for herpes and genital warts. The treatment is remarkably simple. The ozone is produced by forcing oxygen through a metal tube carrying a 300-volt charge.

Planter Warts are cured with silver nitrate are sold at veterinarian surgical supply stores on sticks for about 10$. Wet and apply directly or follow instructions on package. Another method that is not as effective is to apply clear nail polish and apply directly and flair out beyond the edges so as to starve the oxygen to the wart and then cover with duct tape for days. It sometimes works.

Poor is the man whose happiness is dictated by another.

Post dramatic stress disorder

One US soldier is committing suicide every hour every day. Without proof, the troops might be mind controlled through various techniques while in the theatre of war using sophisticated frequencies emitted from fixed and remote transmitters and perhaps intensified by RF micro devices. This might happening through vaccination of all the troops with the injection of the RF micro devices that are so small the computer chips can be injected from the head of the needle. The main emotion desired of the military. One emotion of rage of a soldier is desired when a battalion is sent in to kick the doors open along the streets of peaceful families where soldiers wouldn't normally act this way. It's when they are later discharged and returned home is when the shock and devastation is realized by what crimes against humanity they have committed once out of the theatre of war they were operating under, and back on home soil. Some soldiers shake it off and some don't. I would expect behavior to be on a sliding grey scale. 90% are negatively affected and the worst are committing suicide. I think the negative effects are intensified when the troops realized that the invasion of Iraq and Afghanistan was based on WMD's. We later learned that it was just propaganda without fact. Those who benefitted by having war are the same people pointing the fingers. Look for the signs.

Prednisone

Puts body into stress, by shutting down the brain and the body. It also shuts down the immune system and is a dangerous drug to take for autoimmune because it shuts down the last means of immunity, after autoimmune has taken out the other 2. Prednisone is not a solution for autoimmune patients and is prescribed by doctors who have no understanding of the disease.

Probiotics

You need about 85% good bacteria (aerobic) in ratio to bad bacteria (anaerobic) for optimum digestion, optimum immune system, and optimum mental health, called gut flora. GMO and fast food destroy proper gut flora ratios which can lead to IBS, leaky gut, and pain in the digestion area of the lower right side of your belly.

Prostate cancer

Reversatrol, ambrotose and glutathione will help with prostate inflammation. I believe that taking DHEA might be the solution to prostate cancer. Testosterone should never be taken unless it is opposed to DHEA. A portion of the Testosterone will turn to Estrogen, and unopposed free estrogen along with xenoestrogens found in plastics like BPA and BPS is one of the causes of many cancers including prostate cancer ovarian and breast cancer. My guess is that prostate cancer should be taken with 50mg of DHEA daily to balance out the unopposed testosterone and resultant estrogen and mimickers found in the lining of your beer cans, non-organic laundry detergents and underarm deodorants.

Reiki

REI means universal spiritual wisdom and KI means the life energy. I found both Reiki and Crystal healing to be profoundly beneficial when performed by gifted practitioners. Both focus on the chakras and energy alignments of your body. It is helpful in the initial start of everyone's healing journey because the benefits are immediate. It seemed to give everyone patience of those looking for instant gratification which gave the other elements of health a chance to kick in over the days and weeks after completing just 1 session. Both are solutions for removing unwanted elements of 4th dimension psychic attacks, which are more frequent than people realize. Attacks happen when your frequency gets too low from depression or use of drugs and if your frequency gets too high. I believe that Britney Spears was one such public victim a few years back.

Restless Leg Syndrome

We were able to get rid of restless leg syndrome and arthritis with a high density meal replacement. It takes about 10 days to 2 weeks for nutrient loading and cellular absorption. Leg cramps I found were relieved in a day or two with electrolytes, so try both remedies.

Salt

Is good for you and is essential for breaking down protein into amino acids in your stomach. Salt is an ionic bond and without salt in your body, it cannot send electrical signals properly. Salt should be taken daily and it helps to lower hypertension. It is regular table salt that is toxic and is thought to contribute to plaque formation on blood vessel walls by irritation of those surfaces. Sugar and HFCS are other irritants to healthy blood vessel walls as well. Organic sea salt and better still is pink Himalayan sea salt that are healthy for you.

A Sinner

A sinner is someone who controls another.

Skin

Is a symbol of health and is the last to receive nutrients and it is one of the organs that eliminate toxins. It takes about 10-14 days of nutrient loading in the blood to get benefits out to the skin. Whatever goes on your skin goes into your blood, absorbed through the fat tissue. It is your body's biggest organ. Skin plays a key role in protecting the body against pathogens and excessive water loss. Its other functions are insulation, temperature regulation, sensation, synthesis of vitamin D, and the protection of vitamin B folates.

Spina bifida

Is a birth defect that involves the incomplete development of the spinal cord or its coverings. Like most disease is caused by a nutrient deficiency of the 77 essential nutrient elements during gestation.

Shingles

Relief in minutes came from taking a tbsp. of sesame butter and saturating it with cayenne pepper and spreading it on the site of "shingles". Shingles is caused by a virus and viruses can be suppressed and perhaps "cured" by taking 10 drops of h2o2 a day in an 8 oz glass of water. With the blood oxygenated the virus should die. Viruses hide in healthy cells dormant until triggered by fatigue, malnourishment, dehydration and stress.

Sirens

Of ambulances, fire trucks, police cars and trains in urban areas needs to be looked at. The sirens scare the hell out of people subconsciously and consciously make people depressed and keep people awake at all hours of the day and night as if the end of the world is happening. Sirens are hurting more people than they help. I see the sirens of fire trucks are needlessly used to show up and turn off alarms in apartment buildings. Trains are travelling across the country blowing bull horns you can hear 2 miles away with earplugs in at every crossing from ocean to ocean in every community at all hours of the night. A car horn seems to work for everyone else, but people only use them when someone or something is in the way? Perhaps common sense should be left to the drivers and taken away from Authority.

Stomach cramps and diarrhea

Organic apple cider vinegar, 2 tbsp. in a glass of water gives relief within 15 minutes. Cause usually is GMO's, exposure to mold and stress for some.

Sunbeds

Most tanning equipment uses magnetic ballasts to generate light. If you hear a loud buzzing noise while in a tanning bed, it has a magnetic ballast system and that gives off an unhealthy EMF. Try to avoid magnetic ballast beds and restrict your use of tanning beds to those that use electronic ballasts. They give off more of the healthy UVB than that of UVA light. Sunbeds help reduce acne.

Television

Television is a drug. You can tell if someone is programmed when they stop being critical and stop thinking for themselves. They stop having an opinion from what is different than what is on TV. The televisions have a flicker rate that puts people into a trance after 5 minutes. Pay attention to yourself sometime when you forget that you are watching a show you can't stand, and from out your trance you realize you need to change the channel. Pay attention to the nonsense and fear that makes you feel depressed watching the News.

The Sarin poison gas killing Syrians has orphaned 1 million kids by the Authority who is blaming it on rebels under a false flag event. Our rulers want to use Syria as a staging ground for the invasion of Iran. They don't yet control their bank and want their oil. North Korea is the other remaining bank the 134 families don't control. Watch the Reality Check on the New World Order by Foster Gamble just released.

Thyroid

Iodine with selenium along with B2 to work properly. If in doubt take a triple dose of iodine and work with your doctor to eliminate your thyroid medication. Iodine works slowly and stops women's hair from falling out in fact it makes it go lush and improves your vision acuity (see iodine). 60 minerals found from a Utah sea bed, 16 vitamins, 18 amino acids and the 3 EFA's found in meal replacement helps with all cellular function in the body.

Toe Nail Fungus

Soak your toes in Listerine mouthwash to rid of toenail fungus. The powerful antiseptic leaves your toenails looking healthy again.

Toothache

The main cause of toothaches is exposure to toxic mold. If you sleep or work or vacation in a moldy space that smells musty watch for the signs. Toothaches are a sign of exposure to toxic mold, but might not necessarily go away once removed from mold. A mold-free environment should make root canal far less common by recognition of the cause.

Toothpaste

Calling poison control is suggested if you digest a pea-sized amount of toothpaste. Fluoride is a toxic component and should be avoided by using organic toothpaste. Baking soda makes for the safest and most effective toothpaste or toothpaste from a health food store is a must.

Tylenol

Is the leading cause of liver failure in America. Acetaminophen is a very toxic substance to reduce headache and pain. Headaches are primarily caused by inflammation of somewhere else in the body and or toxins. Pain and inflammation is a major cause of depression.

Vaccinations

From what I am reading from scientific research, is that vaccinations have never been proven to work and increase the likelihood of getting the disease it was meant to protect. In an interview with Merck vaccine scientist Dr. Maurice Hilleman which was recorded, (you can find it on Youtube.com under the videos by vaccine enthusiast Dr. Len Horowitz), admits that vaccines contain dozens of hidden cancer viruses derived from diseased monkeys along with the presence of SV40 and AIDS in vaccines. Tens of millions of Americans have been injected with this contaminated polio vaccine that the CDC is currently trying to sweep under the rug.

Vaccinations seem to result in a soft kill of babies, by way of damage to their brains and the rhythm of life. 25 vaccinations are combined in the 1st 2 years of a baby's life. It destabilizes the body, and rewires the immune system. Why would you squirt 50,000 units of mercury into a child where 1 unit is toxic? The mercury is disguised as thimerasol on the side of the box. The brightest kids seem to be the most affected. Severe autism 100 years ago used to be 1 in a 100,000 and now it is 1 in 50. I believe that the autism rate is 100% of all children who are vaccinated. The frequency, the light in a child's eyes deaden, IQ's seem to drop following a series of vaccinations. Taking vaccinations cause inflammation in the brain and throughout the body and destroys natural immunity.

A researcher did a study of 19,000 children and the response back from parents were that the children who were vaccinated were 4 times or 400% more likely to be sick than kids who weren't vaccinated. h2o2, hydrogen peroxide makes any disease or ailments that vaccination is intended for, irrelevant. Who do you believe, the studies that were bought and paid for by the Pharmaceutical Companies or non-partisan doctors trying to warn the public? Mercury is the most toxic element there is on earth, there is nothing more toxic, but we haven't finished there. They add aluminum to that dose that effectively conducts the Mercury through the blood brain barrier where the Mercury begins to slowly dissolve areas of the brain it comes in contact with. You can see the instant annihilation of the cells under a microscope. Reading the scientists reports from chemtrails, aluminum makes mercury 10,000x more toxic, and the aluminum is toxic itself and if that is not enough the Pharmaceutical Companies add Squalene, a highly toxic adjuvant to amplify the immune response. Because vaccinations bypasses the adaptive immune system the only response possible is an innate immune response to the adjuvant which is dangerous, harmful, and painful. The immune response results in a cytokine storm called an autoimmune response that calls in killer T cells and B cells. 24% of children will be susceptible to an autoimmune disease known as Juvenile Rheumatoid Arthritis which you can predict prior to injection with a HLA-dr blood test done on chromosome-6 looking for a particular subtype. A common subtype is 52b. The rest will be lucky and only experience autism and degenerative brain functions and ADD and ADHD or just a lowered IQ. If you don't believe me ask the mothers who vaccinated their kids and had them screaming following, with varied side-affects that were not healthy and remained that way.

The doctors don't research the contents of the vaccinations and it might be a big part of their compensation and their authority reprimands them if they don't vaccinate. They look the other way and administer the poison without question as loyal obedient servants of the insane directors of the system. Vaccinations are enforced by law in some states as mandatory and not in the interests of their patients. And most doctors ought to know it and should.

Dr. Diane Harper, key developer of Gardasil, admitted that deaths from Gardasil have been underreported by the U.S. *Centers for Disease Control and Prevention* (CDC), which has given the illusion that the vaccines are safe.

The truth about Gardasil and its counterpart Cervarix has been revealed, and still nothing has been done to pull the vaccines from the market. California and Michigan are actually administering these two vaccines to some children without parental consent, and many other states are "mandating" it for students who enroll in public school.

Doctors and parents need to visit www.Vactruth.com and familiarize themselves with the ingredients of what they are squirting into their babies.

The doctors are depending on the pharmaceuticals who are chronically and consistently found to be corrupt, with support and cover up by the media, pretending to be investigative. It's already been proven that the MMR vaccine caused autism in court awards to children taking it. Formaldehyde is a toxic embalming fluid to stop dead people from rotting and is contained in vaccinations and in soda but not allowed in toys. Mind control ingredients are suspected to have been added to vaccinations for the "V-mat 2 gene" that stimulates desire and beliefs and is on a Youtube video.

There are scientific reports out that say there are serious health risks associated with the Tdap vaccines. Also, there are relatively benign health implications that are commonly associated with the diseases the vaccine are intended to prevent, with the important fact from one report, that "vaccines have never been proven to prevent any disease."

Vitamin D and the Sun ☺

Vitamin D is the second most important supplement to health that there is, next to Iodine. It begins to work at a minimum of 5000iu/day and is equivalent to a ½ hour of midday sun. It is a fantastic anti inflammatory vitamin that works better than Advil, Aspirin, Tylenol and Aleve. When taken 5000-10000iu/day it works as an anti inflammatory that has many beneficial health benefits and anti-cancer benefits. People with cancer should ramp up their Vitamin D to 50,000iu/day in a single pill sold in the US, but not for longer than 6 months because there are liver toxicity concerns if left at a high dose. Menstrual cramps go away with 5-10,000 iu of vitamin D within 30 minutes, and taking EFA's for a couple of months helps.

Cancer patients and anyone with a disease and the over weight should get as much sun as possible without burning the skin. Autoimmune patients will be more sensitive to the sun because of low MSH hormone. The midday UVB rays of the sun is the active frequency of healing, and is detoxifying. Make sure you don't burn and make sure you don't wear sunscreen, and if you have to, make sure it is organic. The healing midday sun prevents cancer and alleviates autoimmune disease symptoms and eliminates a few lbs of excess fat through the reduction of inflammation. Sun improves mood and energy levels through the release of endorphins and is good for:

- Melatonin regulation and synchronization of your biorhythms
- Suppression of the symptoms of fibromyalgia and multiple sclerosis and disease
- Treating skin diseases (including psoriasis, vitiligo, atopic dermatitis, scleroderma) and antibiotic-resistant infections, (MRSA) a heavy dose of Iodine is the key supplement for MRSA patients and the disease is primarily a symptom of low iodine.
- Treating tuberculosis, neonatal jaundice, and T cell lymphoma

It is interesting that Health Canada recommended for years 400iu/day and today recommends 2,000 iu max of vitamin D per day when it only begins to work at 5,000 iu/day. Another source of misinformation the department is intended to serve.

Vitamin K
Good for platelets in the blood to stop clotting and for healthy bones. Best taken together as Vitamin A, D, K for balanced absorption.

Water
The highly toxic industrial chemical fluoride is being dumped into our municipal water system along with the antidepressant prozac, heavy metals, radiation and other toxic chemicals. Where fluoride is not added to the water, it is being replaced with another toxic chemical, chlorine. Chlorine is almost as toxic as fluoride, both designed to kill protoplasmic life and humans are protoplasmic. Both are cumulative and both cause a couple of dozen diseases as well as lowering IQ scores significantly.

Environmental Working Group released a report finding human carcinogens in every single municipal water sample tested, from 43 different states across the United States. They found that chlorine and other water treatment chemicals react with organic particles in the water to create hundreds of extremely toxic byproducts, or DBPs which aren't regulated for testing. Some DBPs are 1,000 times more toxic than chlorine or fluoride and include trihalomethanes, which are linked with bladder cancer, miscarriages and stillbirths, disease and inflammation.

These toxins are not necessary if we were to disinfect our water with oxygen. Oxygen is the superior product for the job and only needs 1/5000th the volume to deliver the water alive at the tap to continue killing disease and inflammation throughout your body after you drink it. The more you drink the healthier you get. The more municipal water you drink in North America the more toxic you get, and with iodine bleached out by fluoride and chlorine, the more probability of getting disease you have and the fatter you get!

Thought:

Water is the blood of the earth. Cutting trees makes water lazy by becoming warmer. Shade gives water cooling where it becomes more-dense. At 4C/39F water cannot compress and at 5C it begins to expand. Every artesian well is at 4C, this is the temperature of the purest water in nature. Without water nothing lives. When water becomes warmer, it loses its lifting ability to cleanse rivers. Warm water plugs up rivers. Straight rivers never work. Rocks and bends in rivers give the water a source of energy. It is the flow and coolness that lifts muds and cleanses. It is the spin vortex of fractality that gives water its Life Force energy that can transfer its energy to those who drink it. Water neutralizes stomach acid so it's best not to drink with meals. Distilled water is a hungry water that pulls minerals from your body. Best to add a pinch of plant minerals to neutralize that negative attribute.

Disease is easy to understand and its remedy is repetitive and virtually the same for any disease. There is more than one path to recovery. You need 2 items to get healthy, 6 items to get really healthy and 4 more if you have disease. There are less significant products you can use, that confuse everyone totaling perhaps 50 or 100 that lower inflammation somewhat. They help but aren't necessary. Meal replacements for nutrition, sold in a canister are excellent, but the one I used was awesome. For people who held the products, their hands would vibrate with the energy coming off it. I would like to get the homemade products into production perhaps with donations to get these vital products out to each and every one who asks for them or can't afford.

70% of the US population are living paycheck to paycheck. We need jobs returned and perhaps all those companies that left the US and Canada in the last decade might come back if we close the doors to their imports. We just need to pull the plug on those who make decisions for the benefit of corporate interests, instead of the people they were hired to take care of. They are destroying China now, similar to how they did in the US, by sucking the population off the farmland into the factory jobs located in the cities and buying those stressed farms at pennies on the dollar. Soon those factories will find another home when wages go up and they collapse China's industrial complex but not before the farmland is bought up to control their food supply. China is now drunk on the cool-aid of illusion.

THOUGHT:

Food is a life form. The body doesn't waste anything and operates at 100% potential despite deficiencies. I talked to another doctor today who has a formula on the shelf that with 32 calories in total, from 2 tablespoons of liquid gives an athlete enough energy to run a marathon. The product is fermented in a glass of water and defies the Krebs cycle theory of how energy out of a calorie works. Another product is fermenting platinum to wipe out cancerous tumors, and fermented lithium that is natural and has no side effects to stabilize manic depression. He is one of the doctors who didn't get shot. He got away. There are many products sitting on shelves waiting to come out to the public once assurances of harassment from our government ceases.

Why do guerillas have big nostrils?

Because they have big fingers.

Answer:
You jump into the river and swim across. All the alligators are attending the animal conference. This tests whether you learn quickly from your mistakes.

Chapter 9

The Simple Solution

Everyone deserves to be healthy

Welcome to 21st century. I believe that there should only be one rule that everyone gets health care when they need it and for all to access food and clean water absent of toxins full of nutrients. What do you believe, what is your passion?

Your cells lives off nutrients. The less toxins in your body, the healthier you get. Your body lives off nutrients it recognizes, referred to the concept of bioavailability and Life Force energy of each bite of food you consume. That is how life works. More kids know about "Grand Theft Auto and Call of Duty" video games that normalize killing and theft than about life. That is where humanity's priorities are. If I was president, poison would be illegal in food, water, and air the same day. The next day raids would be conducted of those who continued to poison our drink, food and water with poison. Our reality today is, the doctors who are bringing forth latest technologies to get nutrients into the body, and technologies to rid the body of poison are having guns pointed at their heads and being put in handcuffs and thrown in jail or forced out of the country. Corporations who are bringing forth poison in food water and air, are being granted shelf space, patents and tax incentives. It has been going on for decades and it has been ramping up since year 2000.

People are so caught up in the quest for comfort, on a treadmill for more money, more possessions, that they don't step back and realize what is happening. Their kids have come into the world with 200 toxins in their umbilical cords, 75,000 chemicals in the food chain. They are then getting wacked with 50,000 units of mercury (the most toxic substance on earth), along with aluminum that intensifies toxicity 10,000x, along with squalene in the vaccinations that cause 100% autism of all kids that take the vaccinations before the they are 7 years old. The baby formulas are filled with GMO's that mutate negatively a baby's DNA to a point where no one knows where that baby's DNA is going? In that baby formula is fluoride or chlorine that is as toxic as arsenic that is cumulative, lowers IQ 20%, causes arthritis, lethargy, and 20 different diseases including hypothyroidism, breast cancer, cystic breast disease, edema, dry skin, dry hair that later falls out, obesity, diabetes, bone cancer, brittle bones and osteoporosis. In that formula is estrogen mimickers that are 10x more powerful than birth control pills. The kids are then paraded down to the dentist, having their teeth filled with mercury fillings. As their teeth continue to decay underneath the filling, the mercury starts to leach into the blood stream of their bodies through their gums. Meanwhile daddy's pension is getting raided and the bank is at the door to foreclose.

Solving health issues is about solving the Imbalance(s) and not about treating the symptom. Symptoms are strictly to be used for diagnosis and are a source of confusion if they are not. It is 1 or more of the 5 imbalances that lead to inflammation. Not only does the Matrix give you access to the door for the cure for every disease and obesity, but it is also gives you the ability to thrive. The cure for humanity can be written on a napkin. The purpose of this book is about how to thrive. My goal is to get that napkin out to everyone so that the knowledge of true health can be achieved by all, by becoming available to all. Share the napkin of life to all you can. Statistics of everyone who used the Matrix was 100%. 50 million Americans are on food stamps, 50% of the US has chronic illness, 7 million locked up and you wouldn't know it by watching TV that there might be a problem as people like me are waving our hands saying, "over here"! The cheat notes for your napkin to disease are in chapter 1 of the 5 elements of the pyramid and of the sequence. The notes for obesity and wellness are in chapter 2 of the "do's and don'ts".

Hope

The guide to lose weight, is the general guide of "dos and don'ts" of how to get rid of inflammation that leads to unhealthy weight. Once on the highway of health, cholesterol, diabetes, cancer, and just about every disease there is and excess weight have nothing to cling to. The suggestions are not weight loss suggestions but how to embrace health. You will notice that all the "do's" are about embracing health and the "don'ts" are about avoiding toxins. With ultimate health you will not have an unhealthy pound of weight on your body.

Weight is a reflection of health and is an arbitrary number only your body will know that ultimate number because weight also includes a function of healthy muscle. The goal of ultimate weight will be found once inflammation is reduced to zero. Chapter 2 was the list the methods to reduce the symptom of excess weight which is a symptom of imbalances of the Matrix of the 5 elements of health that leads to inflammation, aches and pains, disease and cancer and associated symptoms of dementia, low energy, and lethargy as symptoms of poor health escalate. To understand how problems with health works. You have to look at your health as escalating rather than poor health failing you. Health is like a ladder of life that is a sequence you can choose to ascend if only you knew how it all worked and decided which direction you want to go. If you are on chronic medication or have a chronic disease, you are riding the elevator of disease down with your doctor chasing symptoms. But by embracing chapter 2, you can immediately begin to ride the elevator up as your body feels improvement for weeks and months. Your doctor visits will tail off only as you get permission to get off the drugs you have been taking for years.

When the level of one's health falls, the rocks of disease and unfortunate life experiences expose themselves. By raising overall health using the 5 elements of the Matrix, those exposed rocks can submerge safely below an elevated level of overall health. The exception is that health problems you are born with, you will die with. You cannot treat diabetes because it means you still have diabetes you must get rid of diabetes by embracing health. You will still have susceptibility to diabetes but will be safe as long as your health is elevated. This is what they call remission, but remission really refers to a rock(s) in the bottom of your aquarium where the level of water represents your health. Everyone in health care is looking at the rocks of disease or "ill health" and ignore raising the water level of health to submerge those rocks. My point is: "instead of looking at diabetes, disease or weight gone, it is your level of health that needs to be up to achieve a resolution of those issues". Symptoms are just a report card of poor health. You can take out the flower of disease but you must change the soil in which the flower of disease grew. The soil being your health. This book is about reaching your potential of health to the point of thriving well beyond disease and only your body knows where to go and it can be achieved by following the information in the book. Ultimate efforts yields ultimate results. You should get rid of your aching back, chronic headache, low energy, foggy memory, irritability, and perhaps increase eyesight clarity, dexterity, libido, robust energy after finishing a day's work and assume a happier disposition in life with a promotion as well? Only your body knows, the suggestions contained will increase that probability and your self-help and motivational books will begin to make more sense if when you read them you are absent of brain fog and headaches with energy to get off the sofa and act on some those good ideas presented in those books!

Common Sense

Over 90% of people with cancer go through with the "sick care" recommended chemotherapy, which is an oxymoron because it has nothing to do with therapy. It treats a toxic condition with toxins. Despite this abysmal statistical failure, patients still follow the herd mentality of the sheep. You are more likely to do the wrong thing in your health care choices if you do what everyone else is doing, and the statistics prove it, and the by following the money confirms it. Belief is the hardest part to recovery for over 99% of people I met. Curing disease is easy, that is just a day on the calendar. It was trying to get people to believe it!

The innovators and early adopters that cure their disease with nutrition, cleansing and hormone replacement will need to tell others so the suffering of many can come to an end sooner. The only choice that health care offers doesn't work for disease. It works for the drug companies. I was open minded to finding an alternate way but most people are not. My concern is that these alternate ways are currently being eliminated as our governments directed by the drug companies and Authorities, act like cats swatting each mouse of hope dead off the shelves of what we can use to cure ourselves. Oxygen, liver cleanses, meal replacements, vitamins, raids and audits on doctors and of vitamin and nutrient manufacturers, access to hormones, access across our borders through customs are being shut down to vitamin

D and all sorts of healthy methods to eliminate inflammation and disease. This is an abbreviated list and is of urgency. The media that is controlled by Authority is turning a blind eye to reporting facts and the nonsense needs to stop through awareness and talking about issues that are not in the interests of the community we live.

Truth is a word that is absent in our society and we need to rediscover truth. It's going to take compassion for that to happen.

Successful treatment for cancer using MMS, Dr Gerson, Dr Hoxsey, Dr Burzinsky, Black Salve, Laetrile (B17), Dr Rife, Dr Hulda Clark or operation of clinics that practice these methods will get you thrown in jail in the US and Canada. Dr Burzinsky is the latest casualty to be persecuted, with a proposed fine of $400 million with 300 years in jail for curing people of cancer in the US, the land of capitalism and freedom. With no convictions after 10 years of multiple jury trials by the FDA is was freed. Tell me how that is working for you, or helping citizens? The cure for autoimmune disease has been sitting on a doctor's desk in the US for 15 years he can't implement that was proven with 10,000 patients with the FDA breathing down his neck. His cure is not available to anyone. This doctor has the cure for 170 diseases 100% on 10,000 patients for the past 15 years and he is in handcuffs with duct tape on his mouth, so-to-speak. Meanwhile patients are having their intestines cut out of their stomachs right now that don't need to. By taking 2 grams of Olestyr 4x/day on an empty stomach for 2 weeks, preferably 4 weeks means no surgery. If we had a choice absent of authority we would have millions of autoimmune, and cancer patients, healthy and enjoying life right now with body parts intact without missing a day of work. These diseases don't need to exist. I'm not interested in talking about it, I'm interested in "doing". There are over 700 liver transplants a year in one hospital in the US and over 99% don't need to be performed. But the vast majority of our population is being herded onto surgery tables trusting a system and government that has no regard for humanity. Appearing to care is just an illusion. Perhaps getting toxins out of the food, water and our brains causing inflammation, obesity and disease, will make people realize that we can thrive with a lot of changes by embracing the truth with honesty and compassion.

I would like to apologize to anyone I have not offended. Please be patient. I will get to you shortly.

Lawyers are graduating from a program into a system where justice is served to the highest bidder. MBA's graduate trained that, "money at all cost", regardless of people or community is right the right way. We have confessions of lead scientists who developed vaccines, admitting that the formulas hurt people and don't work. We have a confession from a scientist who helped develop Morgellons disease thinking it was to hurt the enemy. It turns out that humanity is the enemy. All these professions, that are not serving the community by design and not by choice, feel that by their participation in the system on their way to a good life, can redeem their souls by giving to charity at the end of their careers or lives. These are the charities where just a tiny fraction of the money collected goes to help the cause they represent, some less than 1% and the average is just 4%, as uncovered by CNN and the newspaper in Florida.

Let's continue? Politicians are nothing more than actors that are more corrupt than bank robbers. Any man with a brief case can steal more money than any man with a gun. The Pentagon's own auditors admit the military cannot account for 25 percent of what it spends. Watch Donald Rumsfeld's acting performance on Sept 10, 2001 the day before 911, where he sadly states that "$2.3 trillion US dollars has gone missing" announced from the Pentagon that got hit, that left a paper trail back to building 7, the 3rd tower that went down the next day on 911, 2001. Rumsfeld is our man who got aspartame approved after years of rejection. Watching Washington operate is like watching a soap opera where the scripts are written long before the performances. These guys are academy award winners rehearsing passion without living it, as if they are trying to get something done with care for the people they serve. The vertical integration of corruption and collusion is so massive and global, it takes at least a year to comprehend, and only after every detail is laid out for you.

Youtube.com "Max Igan, The Calling" to get started and later try the advanced version of, "Esoteric Agenda". Once you learn the facts, it's not hard to figure out where the money is going.

Report on Health Care

If we had the authority we could clear out most of any hospital within a few weeks and the stragglers within months, flushing healthy patients out the exits and a drastic reduction of patients coming in the entrance would save Canada $100's billions annually and you could multiply that amount by 10 for the States and perhaps by 100 for the world. Do you think that might save you some insurance premiums, taxes or lost time at work?

The 5 elements can be summed up into equations:

```
         O                          O
       / | \         vs           /( )\
       ( )                          |
       _| |_                       _| |_
```

Neurotoxins In	vs	Neurotoxins Eliminated
Sourced from mold in your home, work and where you vacation		Remove yourself from mold, get max sun and take Olestyr 2 gram/4x/day or less effective Bentonite 2x/day on an empty stomach.
Hormones natural	vs	Balanced and supplemented after age 40
Empty Nutrients	vs	Nutrient Density and Bioavailability
Calories and waste		Life Force energy of food

Toxic Loading In food, water and air	vs	Toxic elimination from cells and organs by cleansing and body's elimination over time.
Inflammation = low energy Depression, low frequency	vs	Thriving attaining full potential and abundance
Antidepressants, antibiotics, Vaccinations, disease, chemo, Fluoride, Inflammation	vs	Oxygen, Hydrogen peroxide food grade, or MMS, Boron by doctor ND, hyperbaric chamber, or h2o2 IV from a natural path, daily oxygen 11% from a Health food store.

The use of the Matrix and sequence to disease makes disease, obesity, medicine, elective surgery, mental illness and apathy virtually obsolete. I went from an invalid needing help to roll over in bed to eat, to a place of euphoria using information that completely contradicts the current standard practice of health care and not only for myself but everyone else who has tried. The skeptics who verbally express doubt should spend their efforts explaining to me why science said/says cigarettes, Thalidomide, asbestos for insulation, lead for plumbing pipes, aluminum wiring, mercury fillings, are good for you. There is no controversy with ethical scientific results or common sense. Where are the scientists today who profited by saying smoking calmed you and was good for you? How did they profit? Ethical scientists and doctors are speaking out via the internet on these subjects producing horrifying evidence about GMO, vaccinations, chemtrails. 97% of scientists say that global warming is nonsense not supported by science and the other 3% are either stupid or corrupt. Unethical scientists need to go to jail along with the bankers. You have 3 million homes in the US in foreclosure. Do you think it was by accident? Do you think bankers are stupid? That jumbo jet was landed with precision and who profited? Just follow the money.

If you control the market, it doesn't matter what brand you sell it under.

The scientific community and law system favors the company with the most money and not what is in the best interests of the people it serves in the community. If North American society could evaluate data of high rates of cancer and auto immune, interest in these geographical areas could be highlighted and prevention could be rationalized. Cancer doesn't exist around the world in several societies. We have the technology and doctors to regrow limbs and eliminate quadrapalegics in the US. Is anyone interested? Does anyone care? Where is the media?

The doctors are exceptionally trained for trauma care, at stabilizing the patient and acute inflammation. The problem with health care, is that doctors don't learn about resolving problems associated with chronic inflammation that lead to obesity and disease. One has little to do with the other. The propaganda perpetuates itself outward from there. If you want health advice, "ask your doctor". Trouble is doctors learn that disease is arbitrary and solutions are arrived at by consensus among those who are considered health experts. But the truth doesn't care what the experts think. These are the experts who don't have a cure in their tool box to talk about. They are just technicians. The real experts are hiding under their desks like the doctor who can cure autoimmune or those who have fled the country to practice ethical medicine. There is a reason why they are hiding under their desks or fleeing the country.

The chance of having no remedies over the centuries is greater than 1 in a quadrillion times 100,000. There are only 5 elements of health measured by pH. These 5 elements are not in the health books. It's a dog chasing its tail then. The ironic part is that the information on health care in this book came from doctors who are hiding from Authority. Authority is in the process of shutting down the internet for those of us who have information to share that help people. We need your help and there are brilliant scientists and doctors ready to put forth their solutions without risk of threat or imprisonment.

Eugenics is now called "Planned Parenthood". The higher your inflammation, the lower your IQ, the lower your energy, the higher your cholesterol, the worse your diabetes, the worse your immune system, the higher your depression, the higher your dementia, the higher your apathy, the higher your health care costs, the more the absenteeism you suffer, the more back pain you have, the more depression. Some people are more sensitive than others. People are now living in communities like they are in a microwave oven and the electronic intensity is ramping up without regard for health. Authority knows the resonant frequency to kill your immune system, fertility and that is what you are getting every day. What changes or advancements for the better have you seen in the last 20 years to prevent disease or improve health? Actions speak louder than words.

There are 4 new sources of toxins newly intensified in the last decade as electronic smog (smart meters, smart phones, wifi, flat panel television, TV games, cordless home phones), vaccinations, GMO's, and geoengineering that are destroying immune systems, fertility, inflating the problem of inflammation, all interfering with DNA that are promoting cell mutations and thought patterns and ability for people to think. This is happening along with the intensification of ever increasing toxins in food and fluoridated/ chlorinated water and with the elimination of nutrients from our food using state of the art laboratories and engineering.

I think that it's best not to judge anyone until you have walked a day in their shoes and if they haven't got any consider reaching into your pocket and buying them a pair. Perhaps that person probably has something to teach you, that you can't learn from a book. Perhaps they were just more sensitive to the toxic poison in their food, or the pedophilia in their home was overlooked by Children's Aid with no moral oversight or compassion? What is your passion? What do you believe? How can you help?

The psychopaths are running the insane asylum

Thomas Jefferson 1762-1826, warned about centralization of medicine. He said, "If you limit people's ability to access healthcare freely, you can control the people." This is what managed health care is about. Thomas Jefferson also said, "if people let government decide what foods they eat and what medicines they take, their bodies will soon be in as sorry a state, as are the souls of those who live under tyranny" today.

In the past the ruling governments burned books on healthcare and prevented information from getting to the people. I witnessed more than one doctor's license being taken away and put on Quackwatch.com and placed in shame instead of honor. I witnessed other doctors being silenced or forced to leave the country to practice health care. Microbiologists for no particular reason have the highest "suicide rates", most hanging in a closet and the rest having "accidents".

Solutions

- I believe that poison must be removed from food and water and made illegal to be in it.
- I believe that a Life Force index be established and labeled on food and drink.
- I believe that GMO must be made illegal and the crops burned based on ethical science.
- I believe that politicians need to start acting in the interest of citizen's best interests.
- I believe we will need to appoint someone like Ron Paul who has the citizen's interests at heart.
- I believe people need to become healthy for there to be change.
- I believe people need to find passion and desire to ever expect a right to access real health care.
- I believe that when the Power of Love overcomes the Love of Power the world will be at peace.
- I find it strange that there is no law that says that doctors have to cure patients if there is one available
- I find it strange that if a doctor does cure a patient that is not approved he will lose his license
- I find it strange that there are no successful cures practiced by the medical community after 100's of years of searching for one.
- We need a leader today, not a dictator

If you tell a lie loud enough and long enough, the people will believe it Adolph Hitler

Pills start where the symptom of pain and weight gain are ignored and your real problems begin if you ignore the imbalances that caused them.

Your health becomes like that of a pinball game where they whack your ball of life from their note pad of prescriptions trying to keep your ball of health in play. But disease and obesity are an option today. Ideal weight is usually the weight you are not. The ideal nutrient is the one you are missing. Follow the protocol of the weight loss in chapter 2 to find your ideal weight and disease prevention.

You can experience the exhilaration of health using the principal of Life Force energy of the food you eat absent of toxins expressed as a mathematical equation borrowed from the study of fractal science. The universe is a fractal series of singularities. What the scientists realized is that there is really only one thing in the universe. We are made up of the same stuff. All the information of the whole universe is available from the same point and can be accessed by a state of enlightenment from inside ourselves referred to as the heart, because we are part of the fractal series of the infinite singularity as one. This is the basis of science, and the understanding of health.

Freedom of speech includes the right to freely share information with others without interference or threat from the state. But this constitutionally protected principle is under attack in a growing number of states where state licensing boards are increasingly restricting right to speech and limit it only to those who first receive permission from the government to give it. And they aren't giving it. Dr. Cooksey is fighting for his right to disclose how he beat diabetes but he is not the only one being harassed by state licensing boards for speaking his mind. Dr. John Rosemond recently received a cease and desist letter from the Kentucky Attorney General's office for an article he wrote that was published in a Lexington newspaper. I found the laws they make are arbitrary to suit corporate interests and not patient well-being. The only thing more outrageous than a dumb law is someone who enforces it. Their laws are arbitrary, self-serving and criminal because the result of such laws hurt people. Because the hurt committed is on a massive scale it is a crime against humanity. These official agencies are actively committing crimes paid for by the public they are serving. Choice must be available to consider ideas of another whose intent is to help others.

Morality is doing what's right regardless of what you're told. Obedience is doing what is told regardless of what is right.

Doctors are obedient and compensated generously to protect drug patents. They are dismissed if they expose the truth. Today it is "intelligent" to be skeptical but that is just plain dumb, because there is no risk analysis being completed, and that results in "inaction". Doctors don't understand autoimmune except for one, and his age is approaching retirement. Surely the drug patents are up and room can be made for this one genius to come forth? You know something is wrong when 80% of oncologists wouldn't take chemo and you have to wonder about the other 20% who would.

Summary

I believe that change takes a lot of work but will be worth it. If we leave the evil food and drink on the shelves to rot, it won't have a reason to exist. Money is a form of energy. Love is energy. Music is energy. Health is energy, and if you want to pursue energy, you do it through the Life Force energy of the food and water you consume absent of toxins including your environment of where you live and work.

Life begins with nutrition, earth's gift to those who walk it.
Compassion and kindness is about giving, it's what the earth does.
The earth receives her gift of energy from the sun.
Love is the air in your tires that makes the world go around.
Creation begins with orgasm.

Life ends with rage, and with hatred,
Life ends with toxins,
It is the sugar in your gas and the metal filings in your engine oil.
Life ends with war.
It's time for humanity to choose now.
Which do you choose?

To the readers and all,

I am not authorized to advise or help anyone pertaining to the information contained.

Authority has given itself the right to do that. The suppression of ideas to preserve the existing status quo of obesity, sickness and disease can continue to flourish unabated for corporate benefit and not for the interests of the community it serves.

Ideas in this book are just points to consider on your path to wellness and enlightenment. This is my story and everyone's recovery can be different in their responses to the protocols I used for myself. The subject matter is for discussion purposes only for helping humanity realize that health care in the developed world does not exist and a new future going forward still needs to embrace the idea of treating the cause of disease and not the symptoms with the realization that nutrition gives life and that toxins kill life, a concept society and the medical community hasn't quite realized yet. When that begins suffering of humanity can begin to end. Many successes discussed have not been FDA assessed or peer reviewed. My belief is that this is our future of health, ideas of which are much different than the current standard. The law states that only your doctor can treat any medical condition or disease. The law also states that a doctor does not have to use any known cure to treat a disease and the FDA arrests all doctors who do. My opinion from my experience states that if your problem has anything to do with inflammation, weight loss issues or of disease that you should run. Asking your doctor to help cure your disease is like taking your car that needs a tune up to an auto body mechanic. Both are skilled but you are asking the wrong mechanic for help. Until you experience, you won't understand why. Please be well and help others to do so. Choosing wisely is a personal choice you must make for yourself! If your choice doesn't work, reread :)

Public Notice:
Due to recent budget cuts, the rising cost of electricity, gas and oil, plus the current state of the economy, the light at the end of tunnel has been turned off.

SUMMARY

Why?

Who's making the decisions about health care? Let's make sure they don't make another.

You graduate wearing square black hats with shiny ribbons around pieces of paper with letters now added to your names without understanding why? You live in a state where the more you know, the less you understand. You walk past the suffering somehow believing that you are better. I know this to be true because I walked with you. But I was different in one way. I later experienced torture and suffering along with the people holding out their hands on the sidewalks seeking help for medical problems that couldn't be answered by a health care system where millions before me had sought help and all that was offered was poison, cutting off body parts, radiation and welfare. All the riches I gained from my piece of paper, my square hat and letters behind my name was, wisdom and hope that there might be a better way to understand why?

I started to see the illusion of the great ego we live in associated with materialism and elitism by seeing both sides of the coin. Perhaps "why" has eluded everyone for all that exist in a "civilized society of me". A "me" society that lacks imagination, understanding, and compassion breeds "sickness" as an uncivilized society.

The reason anyone has control over you is because you want something from them

There are a massive amount of people who are needlessly suffering in a system controlled by a few. It is not about the money, it's about control. Money is just an illusion diverting us from the potential, we as humans have never realized. Society is sick. Health care is built on a weak foundation of mostly nonsense and illusion and a free monopoly to hold it there with profits going to those participants who go along with the system. We can salvage diagnostics (not all), anatomy, trauma care and surgery from their current trauma care system pretending to be a health care system. There is nothing we can salvage for disease or illness of the current system of "sick care" except lessons. We currently don't have a health care system to deal with the 5 elements of health that are necessary to achieve health.

Buddhism is explained as one word "Compassion" for self, and of other life forms, of all that is, as one. Enlightenment can be defined by going inside and connecting through stillness of your mind to all points of knowledge that enables you to connect with the truth. It can only be accessed through health. Life Force can be summed up in an equation that is the mathematical expression that completes Einstein's theory of the Unified Field. Access to this knowledge and happiness can be done through yoga, meditation and compassion absent of fear, regret, hatred, jealousy, anger, frustration, control and belief that holds you there. Humanity has tremendous potential it is not realizing and never will, drowned in a belief that embraces selfishness. How can you trust your eyes if your imagination is out of focus. Out the other side is the answer that "we know everything we need to know". The Unified Field is found through health and it eliminates confusion.

CALM your Mind.

Let's do a check:

1. Do you believe that the bank collapse was an accident?
2. Do you believe that bankers care?
3. Do you think that 3 million home foreclosures was an accident?
4. Do you think that justice is served to the highest bidder?
5. Do you think that the current Charities are good?

6. Did you think that Iraq ever had WMD's weapons of mass destruction?
7. Do you think that Iran and N Korea are bad because we don't control their banks?
8. Do you think politicians work for you?

I believe that change takes a lot of work but will be worth it. If we leave the evil food and drink on the shelves to rot, it won't have a reason to exist. Money is a form of energy. Love is energy. Music is energy. Health is energy, and if you want to pursue energy, you do it through the Life Force energy of the food and water you consume absent of toxins including your environment of where you live and work.

Ignorance is bliss but knowledge is power.

"Problem, Reaction, Solution" is how authority moves its agenda. 99% of the population is asleep to the reality that we have allowed authority to guide our consciousness as a people into....

War	Sickness	Poverty	Apathy	Belief	Suspicion
Starvation	Torture	Enslavement	Deception	Ego	Suppression
Debt	Rage	Lack	Fear	Selfishness	Obedience

Control is by fear, apathy, blind obedience, combined with deception, and the illusion of terrorism. It's not about the money. That is just an illusion, it's about control.

Choice

Chance

Change. You must make a Choice to take a Chance or your life will never Change.

Just say "no"

Curing people of disease and obesity is the easy part, its convincing people to say "no" to control who are preventing it, is the hard part. Choice of health care is our right and sacrifice of self is needed for change. For peace, everyone must put down their guns. It is through sustained selfless, and will power. Embrace what is "good" and change what is not. No savior is coming, you are the "one" to demand change. You are your own savior, no one else is coming. Rigid thinking, institutional control and consumerism is part of control by Authority. One ought to be suspicious to all forms of obedience that requires a certain kind of blind submission to authority. Beliefs of New Age and Religion that "externalizes the savior" is part of the system of control. Through love and sustained will power from within to do for yourself to enact change is the only way out. People will kill for their beliefs, but that is not from the heart. Beliefs "not from the heart" put Jesus on a cross who was here to help humanity. The truth comes from within, not what Authority tells you by finger pointing. The problem is belief we have in Authority. We must abandon Authority and fear, only the truth should be "our" Authority. Perhaps pursuit of the "truth" is the answer we are all looking for?

The problem is choice. Do you want this form of control or this form of control? The concept of Democrats vs Republicans is an illusion of choice who both work for the 134 families at the top of the Illuminati pyramid of power. Many of the politicians are members and are appointed as politicians to positions in Congress and the Senate to carry majority votes on issues that don't serve the interests of the community but serve the Agenda of the Authority. "For your safety, for your protection" are the phrases to watch out for. It is their calling card meant to confuse people.

Try saying "no" to the control system, it is the most powerful word. By withdrawing from what is wrong, you embrace what is right. Knowing "why" is the only real source of power we have. Without knowing why, you are powerless. Not a bullet needs to be fired to change health care and bring forth the cures from doctors who are ready with answers. Authority provokes questions about MS and cancer when answers are here now. If we don't change the system that begins with our food and water it will only get worse. People are already starting to drop like flies in North America.

Control is built on rules, the quantity and the intensity of which is escalating to remove all rights to be free and free of suspicion. Compliance feeds the control of the Illuminati and the 134 families are the Authority at the top and below a population that has a, "I don't care as long as I get mine" attitude. Control is through a police state society dumbed down by vaccinations, GMO's, fluoride as toxic as arsenic that is cumulative, and inflammation, and thought is conducted through a brain that is swirling around in a sea of toxins of which the molecular structures we don't understand, that keep us in a state of confusion and conformity without clarity. The heart of their control comes from a place of ill-health of the many. It is the "me first" desires through manipulation, deception and elitism that divides us. Confusion is the source of control.

Books on good posture, and taking a multivitamin, help you cope with poison help you cope with dying. These are just ideas for temporary patches meant to confuse us. If you are going on a road trip across the country, or you want to start an exercise program, are considering surgery or physiotherapy without first changing your oil and being certain your filters are clean, you are divorcing intellect from wisdom. People spend more on their car maintenance in a year than they do on themselves in a lifetime. "Everything good begins with health".

Who

If everything begins with good health, then all that get in the way, need to get out of the way.

If control is built on rules and rules are made from decisions, who are making the decisions?

That research led me to the 134 families that operate and control the Illuminati and our planet. Washington is a separate country inside the US that is controlled by the Crown which is a country inside of London England that controls the world together with the Vatican that is a separate country within Italy. Your taxes in the US and interest charged on money after banking fees and taxes go to the Crown after the US was forced to go bankrupt following the crash of 1929. Every live birth in the US is issued a chattel certificate where parents sign over their rights to their child and the rights of the child as a citizen and the child becomes a chattel against the debt to the Crown under Admiralty Law. Read the fine print of your newborn's birth certificate before you sign your child over to the State. Watch Esoteric Agenda for more of how your world is run.

Nazi Germany is already here in the US, George Bush Sr. announced the plan of "The New World Order" in his speech on Sept 11, 1991. It was a cloaked declaration of war on humanity on national television. His words haunted me with, "we will win". Win what, is it some kind of war? You can see the video on Youtube.

The New World order is the implementation of Agenda 21 now called "Future Earth". You can see the plan engraved on 20 ton granite stones called the Georgia Guide Stones in Georgia USA. It calls for the extinction of 92% of our population down to 500 million and the ones remaining will be under age 44 all from information contained in the 40 chapter book that Bush referenced. These are not conspiracies because the evidence is clear in the food, the water, the vaccinations, the GMO's, Geoengineering in the skies above and the 20 ton rocks. Actions speak louder than words. They have disclosed this publicly, it breaks no Universal Law, and silence is consent. The timing coincides with the earth's pole shift and the subsequent collapse of the energy grid when earth's gravity goes to "zero point" (Gregg Braden engineer and author) in the coming months. The only way to avoid the culling of 6 billion people similar to the Nazi's decimation of 6 million, is by raising consciousness of humanity by embracing health. The 134 families and the Illuminati in the know and not all are, call this the "X-Factor." The whole system is honeycombed similar to the Manhattan Project where 130,000 employees didn't know what the other was doing to build the atomic bombs out in the desert during WW2.

You cannot solve problems with the same level of consciousness that created them.

Humanity is waking up to the illusion we live in, but not fast enough to make a difference.

Human consciousness can be accessed by embracing health that wakes people up and makes them become aware of what the Families call the "X-Factor". The awareness factor collapses the system of tyranny upon itself similar to the witch dying in the Wizard of Oz. There are huge benefits to humanity if this happens, and profound consequences if humanity doesn't wake up to what is happening to them. It is going to be difficult if people can't comprehend the first step of realizing that consuming nutrients and eliminating toxins are the answer to health. Authority can't calculate for this X-Factor and have done everything they can to suppress health by stealth by removing nutrients from all foods sold in a grocery store. They are gone and the science doesn't lie. The strange thing is that humans are doing this mass culling of one another as loyal obedient slaves because there are only a handful of families controlling over 6 billion of us. It's working like the vortex of a toilet flushing. It happened in Germany and history is repeating itself again in the police state of the US and in other countries around the world. To protect ourselves we need to begin by raising health collectively of the police, the military and the border patrols who are blindly and obediently thinking that everyone is a terrorist pointing guns and surveillance cameras and making good people walk through radiation at airports that harm people's DNA. The Authority are clever masters of manipulation. They are our masters of "divide and conquer".

The handful of families control all media and information sources (radio, television, magazines, newspapers, Hollywood, AP news, Reuters), banking and the flow of money, the corporations (that control the natural resources, the weapons to the food on your plate), the shipping, the stock markets, the airports, the medical, the politics (the pollsters, the polling stations), the education, the military, the CIA, revenue services, the central banks (of every country except N Korea and Iran), they are in control, they're it. There is no competition when you control both brands 51% or more. I believe they are the world's terrorists. You won't find the Central banks or the IRS in the blue pages, they aren't government agencies. Most publicly traded companies are controlled by the 134 families, that's why you have CEO's who are just baby sitters, who risked nothing, who invented nothing making $1 billion of shareholder equity by being just managers and some of them pathetic. What happened to Enron, an oil business connected to Halliburton. The baby sitters enjoy a nice lifestyle, get a small percentage cut of a massive amount, and the rest is going to feed the monopolistic takeover by the 134 at the top. You don't learn this in a university and it's the families at the top putting the programs together for universities. The programming is a form of mind control that convinces you that you understand everything there is available. It entraps you in a belief system that is so powerful, that some kill others to protect it. For those in disbelief follow the money. Who controls Halliburton? The past Vice President (not elect) of the US, Dick Cheney was the CEO of Halliburton and still might be as a shadow figure. Follow the money.

Psst...Terrorists are the people who are aware of those 134 Families who control Agenda 21 which outlines the plan for the New World Order in a 40 chapter book.

Syria has the unfortunate position of being next door to the staging grounds for the US invasion of Iran. The Families have led humanity into every war since 1812 and beyond, slaughtering peaceful Native Indians to follow an agenda of control. Iran is next and North Korea is the final country the Families need to take over their banks, seize their assets and move in their politicians for control. Another 15 journalists have gone missing in Syria that wanted to reveal the real truth while Obama, an academy award actor and the media are getting the propaganda machine in motion for another false flag. These flags are serious and hurt a lot of peaceful people. The Families have just about completed the take-over of every significant corporation, resource and country, and of their national banks around the world. Their takeover worked in Cypress but not in Iceland. Iceland refused to conform. Perhaps we could invite a delegation from Iceland to show us how you lock up bankers and politicians that hurt people?

Ask

Why is there poison in your food and water?

Why are we putting deadly fluoride and chlorine along with anti-depressants and heavy metals in our drinking water tested and confirmed in 43 states across the US, when oxygen is 5,000x more effective at killing bacteria and 5,000,000x more cost efficient when productivity and depression of a healthy population are considered?

Why are you getting vaccinated when oxygen makes vaccinations obsolete?

Why has no cure come out for disease?

Why is our government shutting down access to h2o2, liver cleanses, meal replacements, organic food and supplements? Why are they shutting down vitamins that can save lives?

Why are they putting guns to the heads of Dr. Dahl and his family in Toronto for manufacturing vitamins already approved by Health Canada?

Why is our government telling us that the sun is harmful?

Why are they throwing people in jail for collecting rain water and for making raw milk?

Why are they harassing people for growing organic vegetables in their front yards?

Why are plane travelers having their genitals groped?

Incentive for Change

The clues to the answers are in the movie, The Wizard of Oz where everyone has a brain, a heart, and courage. The soldiers working in the castle are released from their slavery with the death of the wicked witch. It is a mirror image of real life on earth, but there are over 6 billion enslaved. You are currently living in a bad dream where you are led to believe that you have to work hard on a treadmill of debt your entire lives sitting in traffic jams that are by design, stressed to make the next mortgage payment. The few people that make it out of debt slavery are celebrated in the media and held up as carrots for your reward for blind obedience to the system, along with lotteries held up as carrots for those who don't have hope to escape debt slavery. Debt slavery is a form of control that everyone is trying to get out of, even if it means hurting another to achieve. The more ruthless you are, the more you achieve. For those of you who doubt, "follow the yellow brick road."

The yellow brick road represents your gold as money that ends up in the pockets of authority from your hard work. Behind the curtain is the Wizard of Oz who represents our Authority running the system of where that gold or money ends up. The wizard is someone who runs the loyal obedient slaves from behind a curtain using fear and the witch is in your face as fear. But the truth is, that there is nothing to fear. We are living in an illusion that the cure must be found.

The cure for everything has been around for over 100 years, 50 years, 10 years it doesn't matter because it's around, it's here, working now. If you don't believe me, clean your liver, do meal replacement, juice organic, do a few supplements, and watch your medicine cabinet shrink with your waist line, along with life's problems, and your medical premiums.

Misery loves company, but so does happiness

Let's do some math for incentive of our own happiness:

1. Health care costs reduced by 75%, using the cures for disease and obesity that have been found,
2. Sick time reduced 90% by simply making poison illegal and nutrients deemed a priority,
3. Interest charges reduced to 0%,
4. Free electricity - the technology has been around for decades,
5. Free energy for your cars/trucks using hydrogen from water, is available today,
6. Free heat for your house technology has been around for decades,
7. No income taxes, the retail sales tax is enough,
8. $100k for each of you to enjoy.

This is simplified of course but my math says that you could have a 6 month holiday and maintain the same standard of living. You could work 2-3 days a week throughout the calendar and you could still retire much earlier than 65 or 55. You don't need to doubt me you need to follow the money. The major takeover of the US began with the sinking of the Titanic that enabled control of the Federal Reserve by the 134 Families. 600 industrialists, to vote against the takeover, went down with the ship, owned by Rockefeller, a ship equipped with only half the life boats aboard necessary. The women and children escaped and the captain was paid off. The victory was as significant as 911 to move forward an agenda of control. Humanity just needs to place one ethical politician in the White House to unravel the illegal Executive Orders, follow the Constitution, return control of the Federal Reserve back to the people, declare the debts to the Families illegal and declare the war against its citizens over. JFK died trying 3 days after declaring this plan and so have others. It can happen tomorrow, but the chances of returning power back to the people will only increase if you commit to getting healthy.

With 911 they owned the buildings, and the only proof they had that terrorists did it was some lame-duck finger pointing. The proof it was staged from inside was a mountain higher than the towers themselves from information from architects and engineers, camera crews, police, fire fighters, employees from the inside and all without an agenda. 20,000 committed suicide trying to expose that proof. For those in disbelief follow the money. Are those who control Halliburton and the Iraq war tied to the owners of the twin towers? Follow the money for the answer.

Perhaps money could be saved if we could release the prisoners from jail that have never harmed another. I would prefer to put the bankers in their place who have. Choice could become rejoice. Iceland threw their bankers responsible in jail and declared the debts from Credit Default Swaps and the like illegal back in 2008 with no regrets. I wonder if that made the evening News?

Choice

Everything begins with choice. We can never see past the choices we don't understand. Perhaps now we can. What do all men with power want, more power. Choice is an illusion presented to deceive humanity by those who have control. Charities are controlled by those in control having authority. The cures for charity were found last century. Humanity is at war with authority. Everything being introduced in the last 20 years will make you acidic, sick, obese, and diseased; everything being taken away will make you acidic, sick, obese and diseased. Petroleum will make you sick, acidic, obese, and diseased and it exists in every plastic, food, water, shampoo product, and as gasoline exhaust you breathe every day.

Authority is directing humanity to:

- Make vaccines they know don't work and soft kill those who take,
- Plant GMO's they know will destroy your intestines, your organs, and reproductive systems,

- Add a cocktail of poisons and anti-depressants into our drinking water they know are putting people's minds into a brain fog who drink it. The scientists who make this stuff know that it hurts people.

Authority puts a gun and a uniform in the hand of someone and tells them, "there's the terrorist, that's the bad guy". There is a story Sept/13 where Chicago police were called to a situation of a 95-year-old WW2 veteran, John Wrana, who refused to go to a hospital for a urinary tract infection. Called by paramedics to assist, the Park Forest police showed up in riot gear and proceeded to shoot John with a stun gun and then with a bead bag fired from a shotgun. He no longer needed treatment because he died from internal bleeding and blunt force trauma. This is the same Authority that owns the media from top to bottom that are reporting it 3x on the radio now, the TV tonight and in the newspapers tomorrow and in the magazines next month on three different networks at the same time. The result is a police state where harassment is going on like everyone is a criminal, no one can be trusted and the boogeyman is going to get you! Meanwhile Congress and your Constitution don't matter anymore. They don't need to buy those, they just need to bribe them. How do I know this? Because the preponderance of evidence of decisions being made in last couple of decades since I've been paying attention, are hurting people and helping authority. Who benefitted by the 3 million foreclosures, 10 million manufacturing jobs lost and the spin off work from those jobs being sent overseas with tax incentives to do so? Who bought up your pensions and nest eggs in the stock market at pennies on the dollar of those wiped out who couldn't afford to stay invested with jobs lost, along with their health care gone. These are the honest who worked their entire lives approaching retirement and got sand bagged! Control is fed off our energy. Authority is feeding off our energy. We are their battery. Control is sucking the energy out of humanity and the result is misery that is feeding a spiraling vortex down and those that are living in their Ego will not see it. They will see it when their pensions and police pensions disappear. The police and military pensions will be the last to go because they are part of implementing control for Authority.

BUT HOW?

Authority is twisting the truth creating fear and nonsense that is turning humans against each other and has been doing this for 100's of years through wars, started through staged events with trickery and illusion, and they are getting better at it with practice. The UN was created post WW2 to prevent war and there never has been so many incidences of war in the history of the planet since its creation. The creation of the UN was established for the purpose of peace that led to an increase in destruction and more than 260 wars and outbreaks. To achieve peace you have to go to war? People are peaceful. I see it on every street but the media would lead you to believe otherwise. The media just reported that having mercury fillings in your mouth is not a health risk. One part per billion of mercury is a health risk. The average American has enough mercury in their mouths to contaminate a large pond, and some a small lake by standards that are set by the EPA. There are 100's of tons of it loaded into fillings each year by the dental profession. It has to stop.

We are being carpet bombed from chemtrails in the air, poison in our food and water, mind controlled by electronics. It's recently been discovered that $16 trillion has been taken by the Federal Reserve and given away to foreign banks through a form of embezzlement with just a recent cursory audit of a blank check bailout that was issued by Congress back in 2008. We don't have time to prove what's wrong because it is happening so fast. We can barely keep up and need people to wake up by getting healthy. My math says that they just stole $50,000 for every man woman and child in the US, and we owe $50,000 for every man, woman and child to those same people. We could declare those debts illegal. If we were to confiscate the banks and corporations illegally acquired since they took over the Federal Reserve in 1912 that would give each citizen another $100,000. There is a mountain of truth you should investigate for yourselves. Its worth about $800,000 for each family of 4 to do so, and we could make plenty of room for them at the same time in a cell with an hour of play time each day. North Americans worked for this money. First we need to take control of the media from the 134 family's control, so that we could get the word out to the public about the good News, lord knows we could use some.

I wonder if we can elect the politicians from Iceland to clean up our mess? We could be enjoying life with a 6 month holiday on them!

The Solution, World debt goes to zero and we get real health care and free energy!!

To overcome authority we as humanity must truly become selfless opposite of selfish. Tell someone every day that they are beautiful and look at them when you do. Start with your enemies, otherwise humanity will remain as slaves to the system of control and authority without a choice to be healthy or free from debt.

Perhaps we do know everything there is to know?

Anyone with wealth over $100 million dollars could be confiscated and redistributed to others on the planet who have wealth below $1 million. No one needs more than $100 million, and it makes "more room" for entrepreneurs. This plan would mean over $100,000 distributed for each man, woman and child walking the earth. It is the plan opposite of what they did in Cypress in 2013 where the money of bank accounts that exceeded $100,000 was confiscated and put in the pockets of authority of those with assets over a billion dollars each. The 134 Families had the right idea, but they did it backwards. It seems that most things they do is backwards. If we retired what we "owe" them, we could retire mortgages and credit card debt, to the tune of $100,000 for every man woman and child in America or Europe, "poof gone". If you were to follow the money, it has been siphoned off for the past 100+ years. It means that the world's debt is owed to a handful of Families that have high jacked the central banks of the world of each country for control. Success is measured by how many lives they can destroy and business is good. The collapse of 2008 was beautiful, I call the normalization of nonsense!

The new plan will guide us out of:

War	Sickness	Poverty	Starvation
Torture	Enslavement	Debt	Rage
Apathy	Lack	Deception	Fear

Time for Real Health Care

The cure for every disease and health ailment is known by someone on this planet. What is in this book is a sample. Humanity needs real health care and demand that their health be respected. It will reduce health costs by 80% almost overnight. The trick is to eliminate 75,000 toxins from the food supply and leave nutrients in food. Don't accept less and teach others with patience as they awaken. To have unconditional love for yourself, you need to rid your body of inflammation and take care of it. You were given that body to care for and no angels are coming down to do it for you. It's not about belief, it's more about doing for yourself and helping others. I just want to drink clean water, eat good food, enjoy free energy and have cures available to all. When I am at work I want to know that my government is ethical and protecting the interests of the community, not hurting us.

Being awake means being aware and not accepting anything less than unconditional love for what you put in your body, and surround yourself with. Being awake you will have symptoms you will recognize. Fear is one of them. It is fear that makes your body acidic and you need to let go of fear, you have no use for it. You can love fear to death.

Fear takes you out of love and compassion, and into Ego of selfishness, which is mind limiting. Panic is not a place from which to make sensible decisions. Putting people in fear is the least compassionate thing you can do. Pointing a gun at someone or threatening is as far removed from human as one can be, and so is the graduate scientist putting poison in our food and drink or not reporting the crime. The scientists have a fiduciary duty to the community that places a higher level of expectation of honesty to reporting crime working in fields they specialize. "They ought to have known" is how the prosecution begins. If we begin to embrace love and each other, their Agenda 21 will fail, and we get to keep all their money and get rid of the world's debt!! It's a plan worth considering. The Authority are only 134 families that run the world with 2 at the top. The world's debt is only owed to them. You can tear up your mortgage and your credit card debt, your hydro bill, your heating bill and your health care bill and go get healthy for a 6 month vacation on them!

Time to start talking to your neighbors

Children are our hope. Start spending more time with them. Plant things with your children and abandon the television and microwaves. The cherished children will teach you more than you can learn in a university. Love cannot be manipulated with fear when there is unconditional love for the other. Revenge is not a symptom of true love. With symptoms of love you will feel kindness, compassion, caring and an inability to have your heart broken. The most valuable asset humanity has on this planet is love and it is the one least practiced.

Trust and remain open.

Stop hurting people,
Put down your guns.
Please try to heal yourselves,
Please try to help others to heal,
Please try to help humanity heal,
Those of you feeling compelled to help please feel free to.

The reason anyone has control over you is because you want something from them

To the Authority, we don't need your corrupt banks, politics or your corporations. We'll make our own or just change the signs on the ones we have. We'll have Congress vote that there is no debt. Who is going to tell us what to do? We can close the doors to the FDA with its fluoride, vaccinations, and suppression of cures and all that hurt people. Close the doors to Monsanto that make GMO's. By Executive Order, "We the People" hereby declare hurting people illegal. If you feel pain don't ignore it. If you are hired to cause pain, stop. If you see someone causing pain, stop them.

We have to shut down the pain at the source and stop the confusion. We need to take back the White House, Pentagon, The Federal Reserve. "How does it get any better than this?" For those who are worried, we could stop paying our credit card debt, mortgages, our car payments, and taxes for a start and redirect money into the pockets of Americans for a holiday. (see MoveOn.org to start) This can happen for Europe too. Ask yourself, "What is right about this, I'm not getting?"

When it is safe, could then make available healing centers involving autoimmune remedies, hormone replacement, nutrition, cleansing, and loving people to help raise patient frequency. We can set up clinics in any host country to eliminate autoimmune, MS, chronic Lyme and Lyme disease, diabetes, obesity, cancer, cholesterol, high blood pressure and any disease. We need your help to make this happen. Watch the recreation and vacation business explode when we do.

We need lawyers to come forward to start helping groups bring about honest change to a corrupt system.

We need to help our farmers from the bullying of Monsanto.

We can be better off with their doors closed.

We need to protect our human rights from police brutality.

We need to get rid of organizations that are hurting people.

We need to start asking questions of why this is happening.

We need to start serving the interests of the community instead of ourselves.

We have to start caring.

I've learned so much from my mistakes...I'm thinking of making a few more!

Additional Research on Youtube.com, your homework assignment.
Below is the work by people who care.

THRIVE full length movie by Foster Gamble
Reality Check on the New World Order by Foster Gamble - a new movie full of facts
The Truth About Smart Meters - Brian Thiesen
Nassim Haramein - Science behind the Unified Field & Its applications of free energy.
Dan Winter on Fractality and Sacred Geometry - for healthy food
NaturalNews.com with Mike Adams - daily articles and the real news today

Money as debt - animated documentary
In Lies We Trust by Dr Leonard George Horowitz
Dr Rima Laibow on Codex Alimentarius
The GMO Threat Full Length by Jeffrey M Smith
Max Igan the calling - one of the best
Esoteric Agenda - compelling info
Food Inc - If you shop in a grocery store you watch this film
The Matrix Reloaded - Based on fact
http://www.geoengineeringwatch.org/coast-to-coast-am-daily-march-13th-2013-geoengineering-threats - 3 parts to listen to that are compelling, (Www.carnicominstitute.org)
Eceti.org for access to James Gilliland's books - as seen in the movie Thrive
StopTheCrime.net - Download your free 44 page document outlining the post WW2 strategy to use silent weapons to take
Over the country and implement Agenda 21. You can actually read an "official" doc. written 65+ years ago coming true.

THOUGHT

Perhaps women shall be the new leaders of the next century to show us what it is like to live with compassion of self and of others. The men of the last century have been doing a lousy job. Life ends with a bullet and life can thrive with change. The only thing that remains is truth and a world without pain.

Love Life, Hope, Thrive, Help, Inspire, Kindness, Explore, Compassion.

It's your choice whether cures are brought forth. They are here for you when you are ready.
The End.
Or is this the beginning?
The book is meant to assist with presenting ideas that might work and suggest dismissing ideas that don't.

I have been blessed with this information and wish to share with others to help them find their truth to wellness.

I would love your feedback,
Adam Masters.

And as you slide down the banister of your life, may all the splinters point in the right direction. Merrily, Merrily, Merrily, Merrily, Life is but a dream.

Please help spread the message to those that are suffering, or help someone who is.
(Photocopy next page cutout for your wallet to pass along)

GIVE THE GIFT OF HEALTH
Cut out, photocopy & give away

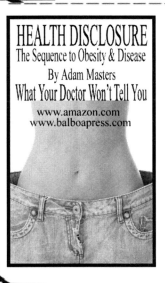

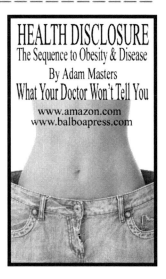

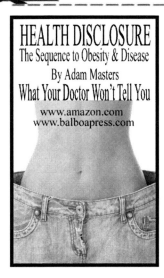

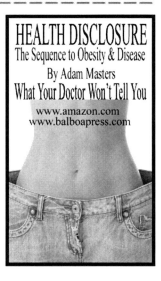

GIVE THE GIFT OF HEALTH
Cut out, photocopy & give away

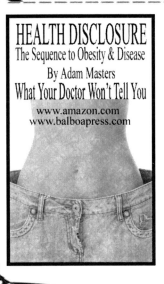

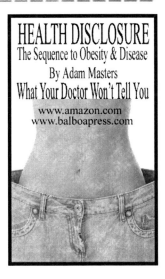

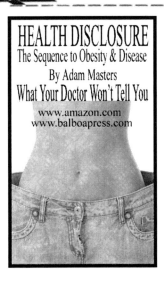

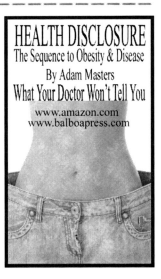

CPSIA information can be obtained at www.ICGtesting.com
Printed in the USA
LVOW06s0625231113

362452LV00004B/19/P